Physical Fitness

Physical Fitness
A Way of Life
Fifth Edition

Bud Getchell
INDIANA UNIVERSITY, EMERITUS

Alan E. Mikesky
INDIANA UNIVERSITY—PURDUE UNIVERSITY INDIANAPOLIS

Kay N. Mikesky
FACTUAL FITNESS,
CERTIFIED HEALTH/FITNESS INSTRUCTOR

Allyn and Bacon
Boston • London • Toronto • Sydney • Tokyo • Singapore

Publisher: Joseph E. Burns
Series Editorial Assistant: Sara Sherlock
Composition Buyer: Linda Cox
Manufacturing Buyer: Megan Cochran
Cover Administrator: Brian Gogolin
Production Administrator: Susan Brown
Production Coordinator: Thomas E. Dorsaneo
Editorial-Production Service: Melanie Field, Strawberry Field Publishing
Electronic Composition: TBH Typecast, Inc.

Copyright ©1998 by Allyn & Bacon
A Viacom Company
160 Gould Street
Needham Heights, Mass. 02194

Internet: www.abacon.com
America Online: keyword: College Outline

Earlier edition(s) copyright ©1992, 1983 by Macmillan Publishing Company
and 1979, 1976 by John Wiley & Sons, Inc.

Library of Congress Cataloging-in-Publication Data
Getchell, Bud.
    Physical fitness : a way of life / Bud Getchell, Alan Mikesky, Kay
Mikesky. — 5th ed.
        p.   cm.
    Includes index.
    ISBN 0-205-19874-0
    1. Physical fitness.   2. Exercise.   I. Getchell, Bud.   II. Mikesky, Alan.
III. Mikesky, Kay.   IV. Title.
RA781.G47   1998
613.7—dc21   97-50489
                                                            CIP

Printed in the United States of America

10 9 8 7 6 5 4 3 2   02 01

To my family—Aline and children Jim and Kathy; Cindy and Mike; and grandchildren Andrew, Alex, Phil, Tyler, and Brianne who all make fitness a way of life.

—BG

To Walter, Joyce, Mick, and Glen for giving us a push, and to Kristi and Shane who keep us moving.

—AM & KM

C O N T E N T S

PREFACE

The fifth edition of *Physical Fitness: A Way of Life* continues this text's tradition of taking a positive, realistic, and fun approach to the basics of being physically fit. Regardless of your past experiences with sports or fitness exercise, you'll find information in this book to help you begin or maintain a program of healthy and enjoyable exercise. With today's sedentary and technology-assisted lifestyles, none of us can take good health and fitness for granted. The way to ensure a lifetime of physical well-being is through regular physical activity.

Over the past twenty-two years, this book has served well as a guidebook for developing a personalized exercise program. It is not a book filled with heart disease statistics or scientific details such as the physiology of how a muscle fiber contracts. Such information, although perhaps interesting to some readers, is not necessary for experiencing the good feeling of being active and in good shape. However, some simple principles of physiology are presented to help you understand how your body responds and adapts to stimulating exercise. An awareness of these basic principles will help you set up an exercise program that works.

Let's not kid ourselves: it takes effort to get and stay in shape. There is no magic program or easy way to be physically fit. However, fitness exercise does not have to be punishing exercise. You need to work out hard enough to challenge your body, but the challenge should be well within your own capabilities. The aim of this book has always been to show you how this can be done. But this book is more than a how-to book; it represents a philosophy of exercise—that being physically fit is a way of life.

This book is meant to be enjoyed. It is easy to read, with illustrations designed to amuse you and to show you the many benefits associated with an active lifestyle. As in previous editions, the presentation is geared for men and women, both young and old, especially those who have limited experience in sports and exercise but who want to become healthy and physically fit. Our bodies were made to be used. Medical research has demonstrated that our bodies do not cope well with too much sitting, standing, and low-level everyday activities. An inactive body tends to lose its healthy functioning over time. It is well established that the human body thrives on stimulating exercise. In fact, the 1996 surgeon general's report clearly states that physical inactivity is a major health concern in the United States. This book will help you get involved in an enjoyable and rewarding program of exercise.

This edition continues to emphasize and recommend activities that vigorously challenge the heart, lungs, and muscles. New and updated material has been added throughout this revision. "Way of Life" boxes in every chapter summarize important fitness tips. Each chapter, as in past editions, opens with an introduction and a listing of major concepts to be covered. Key terms are bold-faced in the text, and listed and defined at the end of each chapter. A complete glossary is found at the end of the book. Additional readings are listed at the end of each chapter in the "Way of Life Library."

The early chapters explore the key principles of health and the role of exercise in health and wellness along with the basic components of physical fitness. The initial emphasis is on understanding and evaluating your present physical fitness so that you can begin setting up a workout program that is reasonable, regular, and effective. The basic principles involved in planning a personal exercise program are explained in Chapter 4. Chapters 5 and 6 explore many approaches to developing your cardiorespiratory fitness. Chapter 7 has been updated and expanded to assist you in developing muscular strength and endurance. Chapter 8 is devoted entirely to discussing flexibility, an important component of physical fitness. Chapter 9 provides updated, advanced methods of training for those aspiring to greater goals such as participating in triathlons and regular sports competition. The final chapters deal with related concerns such as nutrition, weight management, heart disease, pregnancy, osteoporosis, injuries, and the environment.

The information in this book is based on the authors' personal research and involvement in directing exercise programs for people of all ages. We also are indebted to the many exercise friends and research colleagues who have contributed to the body of sports medicine and exercise knowledge. Most important, we must thank the many people who have participated in our programs. The involvement of these people has aided us in learning about exercise programs that work—programs that not only get people exercising but help them become committed to a lifetime of healthy activity. We would like to thank the following reviewers: Lynn Darby, Bowling Green State University; Forrest Dolgener, The University of Northern Iowa; Todd Purdham, Catawba Valley Community College; Carol Ryan, North Dakota State University; Donna J. Terbizan, North Dakota State University; and James Zarick, Guilford Technical Community College.

Finally, appreciation must go to the people at Allyn & Bacon, especially our editor, Joseph Burns, and to production editor Melanie Field, copy editor Tom Briggs, and illustrator Stan Maddock for their assistance, expertise, and encouragement in the writing of the fifth edition.

Bud Getchell, Alan Mikesky, and Kay Mikesky

Bud Getchell, Ph.D.

Bud Getchell retired in December 1996 as Emeritus Professor in kinesiology from Indiana University, Bloomington. Bud joined the IU faculty in the summer of 1985 as the executive director of the newly formed National Institute for Fitness and Sport, a not-for-profit organization located in Indianapolis. His assignment was to help design a state-of-the-art facility, oversee construction, and develop a comprehensive array of program centers. After six years, Bud returned to the Bloomington campus to lecture, assist in expanding current curricula and programs in fitness, and do some writing.

Before coming to Indiana University and the Institute, Bud served as professor and director of adult physical fitness programs in the Human Performance Laboratory at Ball State University. Bud is a fellow in and has served as a member of the Board of Trustees for the American College of Sports Medicine (ACSM). He is a past president of the midwest regional chapter of the ACSM. He holds ACSM certifications as a preventive rehabilitative and exercise program director and as a health fitness director.

In September 1991, Bud was honored in Washington, D.C., by being selected as a Healthy American Fitness Leader. This award is sponsored by the United States Junior Chamber of Commerce, the President's Council on Physical Fitness and Sports, and Allstate Life Insurance.

Bud is a member of various professional organizations and committees related to physical fitness and sports medicine. He has served on the United States Tennis Association's Sports Science Committee, the Indiana Governor's Council on Physical Fitness and Sports, and the Executive Board of the National Fitness Leaders Association. He lectures extensively at research, medical, physical fitness, and wellness meetings and was an invited speaker at the second White House Conference on Physical Fitness.

Over a career that spans 43 years, he has contributed to a variety of research, physical education, and sports-fitness publications. He is a co-author of *Perspectives on Health,* a leading health text for high school students. A former collegiate coach and baseball All-American, Dr. Getchell earned his Ph.D. at the University of Illinois in 1965.

Alan E. Mikesky, Ph.D.

Alan Mikesky is an associate professor in the School of Physical Education, Indiana University–Purdue University, Indianapolis, and director of their Human Performance and Biomechanics Laboratory. He also has an adjunct appointment with the School of Medicine, Department of Anatomy, and serves as research associate at the National Institute for Fitness and Sport in Indianapolis. Alan received his B.S. in biology from Texas A&M University and his M.S. in physical education with a specialization in exercise physiology from the University of Michigan. He received his doctorate in anatomy/cell biology from the University of Texas Southwestern Medical Center at Dallas, where he studied the adaptations of skeletal muscles to heavy resistance exercise. He is a fellow of the ACSM, has served as fitness editor for ACSM's quarterly newsletter, "Fit Society," and is a member of the editorial board for the National Strength and Conditioning Association's *Journal of Strength and Conditioning Research*. His current research focuses on strength training for older adults and its effects on changes in gait, balance, incidence of falls, joint proprioception, functionality, and the progression of osteoarthritis.

Kay N. Mikesky, M.S.

Kay Mikesky has been a fitness professional since 1977. She received her bachelor's degree in physical education and French from Miami University (Ohio), where she competed in intercollegiate swimming for four years and danced in the University Dance Theater. After teaching high school physical education and coaching diving and gymnastics, she attended the University of Michigan, where she received a master's degree in physical education with a specialization in exercise science. Kay served as associate director at Dr. Kenneth Cooper's Aerobics Activity Center in Dallas for five years and became the first fitness center director at the National Institute for Fitness and Sport in Indianapolis. She now acts as a fitness facility consultant, personal trainer, and workshop leader through her company, Factual Fitness. Kay is a certified health/fitness instructor through the ACSM and has conducted fitness classes and workshops in Japan, Switzerland, and South Africa.

CHAPTER 1

Physical Fitness and Wellness

This is a book about you. It is a book about managing and maintaining a healthy level of physical fitness. While most people know that regular exercise, along with sound nutrition, is good for their health, they do little or nothing about it.

The biggest hurdle is finding the time. This book will teach you the basics of exercise and ways to incorporate them into your busy daily schedule so that ultimately they become a way of life.

This chapter introduces you to the what's and why's of fitness. In the chapters to follow, you will learn not only about exercise and its benefits but also about how to structure a personal exercise program that is safe, reasonable, effective, and, most important, rewarding and fun.

As you read this chapter, keep these statements in mind:

- In the past, health meant only absence of disease. Today we have a much broader perspective and consider physical fitness to be a key component of total health.
- A recent surgeon general's report highlights inactivity as a nationwide health concern and emphasizes the importance of regular physical activity for improving and maintaining healthful living.
- The modern lifestyle fosters poor physical fitness because technological advances have eliminated much of the fitness-producing physical exertion from everyday activities.
- Everyday activities, even for the laborer, no longer adequately stimulate the heart, lungs, and muscles to produce physiological benefits.

- Society, especially the corporate world, is beginning to recognize the importance of health promotion and the role of exercise in developing and maintaining good health habits.

- Being physically fit means living at your fullest physical potential. Physical fitness is the capability of the heart, blood vessels, lungs, and muscles to function at optimal efficiency. It provides a basis for living a full and rewarding lifestyle.

- The basic health-related components of physical fitness are cardiorespiratory endurance, muscular strength, muscular endurance, flexibility, and body composition.

- To be physically fit does take effort (yes, some sweat), but exercise does not have to be punishing for you to develop and maintain physical fitness.

- Regular and vigorous exercise of the total body is a necessary ingredient of muscular and circulatory fitness—the key to good health and well-being.

Health: To Live Better Rather Than Longer

Most dictionaries define **health** as "the general condition of the body or mind with reference to soundness and vigor . . . the freedom from disease or ailment." Health includes physical, intellectual, emotional, spiritual, and social components. Therefore the degree of health is contingent on the varying states of its components. **Wellness** is "optimal health," in which all five components have reached the highest level. The opposite of wellness is death. As Figure 1.1 shows, health is a varying state with death and wellness at its extremes. This concept is known as the health/wellness continuum. Our level of wellness changes from day to day throughout life depending on the state of each component. Due to sedentary lifestyles, the physical health of many Americans lags behind the other components. Therefore, on the continuum, these people are "just getting by." Fitness and health experts generally agree that regular exercise is essential in the pursuit of wellness. (For more in-depth reading on the topic of wellness, refer to A Way of Life Library at the end of this chapter.)

Being physically fit does not guarantee your health, but it can be the basis for a fuller life. The effort it takes for you to be physically fit can be a sound investment for future health and happiness. A question you might ask yourself is, how much exercise do I need to realize some health benefits? Perhaps you are concerned only about living longer. A recent study by Dr. Steven Blair and his colleagues at the Cooper Institute for Aerobics Research indicates that even a little exercise appears to protect people from premature death. Blair's study analyzed data on 10,224 men and 3,120 women who were classified as healthy.

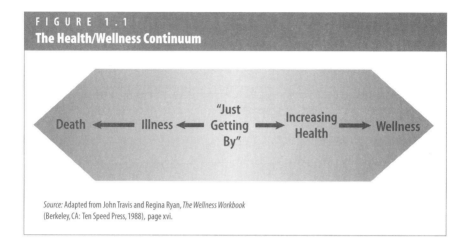

FIGURE 1.1
The Health/Wellness Continuum

Death ← Illness ← "Just Getting By" → Increasing Health → Wellness

Source: Adapted from John Travis and Regina Ryan, *The Wellness Workbook*
(Berkeley, CA: Ten Speed Press, 1988), page xvi.

Based on their treadmill testing results, the participants were divided into five groups, ranging from least fit to most fit. The research team followed these people to determine how their level of physical fitness related to their death rates. After eight years, the inactive group (least fit) had a death rate more than three times that of the very active group (most fit). However, the most interesting finding was that the death rate for group 1 (inactive) was two-and-one-half times that for group 2 (walking 30 minutes a day). Thus the Blair study strongly suggests that even a minimal amount of exercise tends to lower the risk of premature death from heart disease, cancer, and other health-related causes.

Dr. Arthur Leon came up with similar findings in a study that looked at 12,138 middle-aged men. He reported that moderate levels of exercise resulted in one-third fewer deaths among participants from all causes (including heart disease) compared to those who were sedentary.

These studies suggest that minimal to moderate exercise apparently can help you live longer. But is this your goal? Or is your goal to live life to your fullest potential? The classic Paffenbarger study of Harvard graduates looked at the influence of exercise on longevity. Paffenbarger concluded that men who expended 2,000 calories a week exercising lived one to two years longer than sedentary individuals. A case can be made that this is a lot of effort to extend life only an additional year or two. But being physically fit is more than striving to live longer. *Being physically fit is striving to live better.* This is the main theme of this book. People exercise to maintain good physical appearance, to have more energy to carry out everyday tasks, to sleep better, to be able to eat nutritious foods without worrying about weight gain, to improve their performance in a favorite sport or pastime, and, most important, to enjoy the feeling of being physically fit and possessing good health.

Health and Wellness

Recently health professionals have expressed health in terms of degrees (see Figure 1.1). The health/wellness continuum illustrates the broad scope of health from death (total absence of health) to the optimal level of health (wellness). How do you rate your health? Most people would answer "Good" or "I'm fine." If you haven't been sick or visited a doctor recently, you most likely would say you are healthy.

In fact, most people feel that if they are able to carry out their everyday activities, then they are in good shape. In other words, they are not sick. On the health/wellness continuum, such people generally fall in the middle, or "just getting by," zone. They are not ill and may look well, but they may not be especially healthy either. But high-level health and wellness means more than simply getting by—more than being able to attend classes, play intramural sports one or two times a week, work at a regular job, and be active socially. It means being physically active on a regular basis, eating properly, adhering to good sleep practices, and living life with enthusiasm and vigor. Granted, the health risks at the middle of the continuum are not fatal; however, living at a level of "just getting by" robs you of the chance to optimize your health and fitness potential. In fact, nonhealthful behavior over time tends to be detrimental to good health in later life. More important, regardless of age or present position, those who live in the neutral zone of the health/wellness continuum are not living up to their fullest potential. That's the point: What many people have come to accept as "good health" falls far short of what it could—and should—be.

Recently the U.S. Centers for Disease Control suggested that personal health behavior is the major reason for mortality. In other words, your lifestyle is a major determinant of when you die (see Figure 1.2). And a July 1996 report by the surgeon general stressed the importance of regular physical activity for improving and maintaining health and well-being. The report is based on the most comprehensive review of the research literature dealing with physical inactivity and exercise and conclusively links physical inactivity to increased risk for disease. In fact, this report names physical inactivity as a nationwide public health problem. As stated by acting Surgeon General Audrey Manley, "The report is more than a summary of the science—it is a national call to action" to reduce unnecessary health problems resulting from sedentary lifestyles. It is hoped that this report will help catalyze a new physical activity and fitness movement in the United States.

Today more than ever, assuring good health requires you to focus on such health-related behaviors as exercise, nutrition, and rest, to name a few. For improvements in health, we all need to think about changing our lifestyles and personal health habits rather than continuing to rely on modern medicine to keep us well. Keep in mind that health is a mix of factors—physical, intellec-

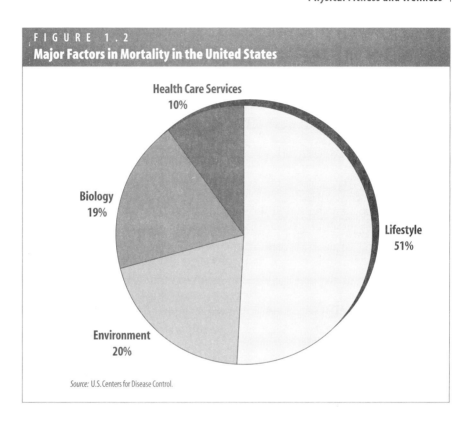

FIGURE 1.2
Major Factors in Mortality in the United States

Health Care Services
10%

Biology
19%

Lifestyle
51%

Environment
20%

Source: U.S. Centers for Disease Control.

tual, emotional, spiritual, and social. Even though you can't control all the factors that determine health, you can take the responsibility for practicing preventive health behaviors. When the first edition of this book came out, we proposed exercise as a key component of good health. Twenty-plus years later, the research evidence unequivocally supports this view. Medical experts now realize that engaging in exercise on a regular basis is one of the keys to health and fitness.

Exercise — The Positive Do!

Exercise is good for you. It can be the "positive do" in your life. Rather than telling yourself, "Don't eat this or that," "Don't smoke," and "Don't get excited," say, "Do exercise." People who exercise tend not to smoke. They tend to be more conscious about what they eat. And they tend to know how to relax. Exercise can be the positive force that helps you adhere to other healthy behaviors. Regular exercise should be an integral part of your lifestyle. It offsets the ill effects of sedentary living in our modern technological society and ensures

WAY OF LIFE
Benefits of Exercise

- Strengthens the heart
- Decreases risk for cardiovascular diseases
- Decreases risk for some cancers
- Decreases risk for diabetes
- Helps to lower and/or maintain body fat
- Improves muscular strength and endurance

- Improves and maintains bone density
- Improves and maintains joint flexibility
- Reduces stress and muscular tension
- Improves quality of life
- Improves quantity of life

that you are living at your physical potential. The benefits of exercise are too numerous to discuss in depth here. However, these benefits will be elaborated on in subsequent chapters.

Later in this book, we will lay out some guidelines for developing a personalized fitness program. Of course, designing a program is easier than actually exercising on a regular basis. But if exercise is fun, you will do it. So what is fun? It's working out with friends. It's setting goals, striving to meet them, and reaching them. It's the good feeling you get from using your body effectively. Fun is not necessarily smiling and laughing all the time. Often people say that they never see runners smiling or that running is boring. But look around you at a concert or a play. Notice that many members of the audience may not be smiling. Does that mean they aren't enjoying it? The point is that fun comes in many different forms. The feeling of accomplishment, the ability to do more things, the sense of energy—all make for a fun life. Living life to the fullest is the payoff for your investment of effort and time in a personal exercise program.

Is Exercise for You?

What are your previous experiences with exercise and sports? Perhaps you have a negative attitude toward exercise. Through no fault of your own, past physical education or athletic experiences may have created this outlook. Experiences such as being punished with exercise, being chosen last in a pickup game, or being ridiculed or feeling embarrassed because of poor skills may have kept you from getting involved in sports and exercise. Punishing

The use of exercise for punishment leaves lasting negative impressions.

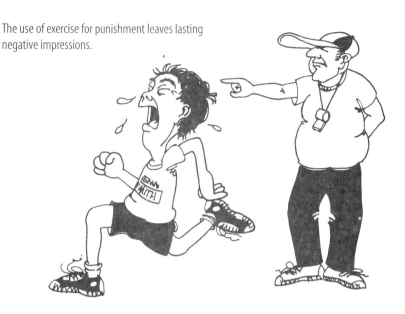

underachievers by forcing them to do calisthenics or run laps is absolutely ridiculous. Allowing an inept performer to be heckled in a physical education class is inexcusable. No wonder so many people do not participate in sports or exercise. Who wants to do something that is associated with pain, punishment, or embarrassment? Obviously not all people can excel in athletics or even make the team. Fortunately, though, physical educators and fitness instructors are now more attuned to gearing programs to individuals' capabilities and limitations than in the past. Regular exercise for everyone is now widely recognized as an important component in physical education curriculums in colleges and universities.

Boys traditionally have been encouraged to exercise and play sports, but physical exertion for girls was long considered unladylike. Today, however, females participate in competitive sports and all kinds of fitness activities. Research now clearly indicates that women respond to vigorous physical training much the way men do. In fact, the research shows that the responses of men and women to vigorous activity are more similar than different.

The American College of Sport Medicine, the American Alliance for Health, Physical Education, Recreation and Dance, and the President's Council for Physical Fitness and Sports all emphasize the need for regular exercise as the basis for good health. Regardless of your past physical education or athletic background, this book is written for you. It provides all the basics to help you discover your own physical resources. And you don't have to be athletic to be physically fit. Traditionally organized athletics have tended to develop superfit competitors for the entertainment of a physically inept society. But programs that reward the best and disenchant the rest leave the majority of people ungratified and even alienated, as well as unfit. Fortunately we now realize that people who will not win championships or even make the team still need invigorating exercise. Why should you be relegated to being a mere spectator? You deserve the opportunity to develop the skills and abilities that can help you enjoy a full and active life. When you feel better as a result of regular exercise and gain a sense of accomplishment by doing something beneficial for yourself, you will become a convert.

Why Physical Fitness?

Although the most opportune time for developing lifelong fitness habits is in childhood, it is in the late teens and early twenties that men and women develop a fitness consciousness. At this stage in life, you have reached physical maturity; your body is at its natural peak of physiological efficiency and health. However, observe friends in their late twenties and early thirties. For many of them, this natural fitness has begun to disappear. Lack of exercise is beginning to show its effect. An increase in body fat, a loss of muscle tone, and a diminished energy level are some of the obvious signs of physiological deterioration. These middle-aged characteristics begin to reveal themselves in many Americans in their mid-to-late twenties. Unfortunately our bodies are not programmed to withstand the effects of inactivity.

Our modern lifestyle fosters unfitness. Many technological advances are intended to eliminate physical exertion from everyday activities. The automobile and television are key contributors to our sedentary lifestyle, and we have become accustomed to other automated energy savers as well: elevators, escalators, riding lawn mowers, motorized golf carts, snowblowers, and various remote control devices. And the 1980s brought us the home computer. Such advances enable us to carry out our everyday chores more easily. Microcomputers not only enable us to keep our home or business records in order but also provide hours of entertainment playing computer games or surfing the Net. However, the rapid, repetitive movements required to manipulate the controls do little for physical fitness. Working out regularly to maintain a healthy level of fitness enables us to enjoy the modern conveniences without suffering the associated health implications.

Overeating, TV watching, and laziness are all detrimental characteristics of a sedentary lifestyle. At the same time, we live in a competitive society characterized by pressing domestic demands, business obligations, and deadline tensions. Smoking, alcohol consumption, and drug use are all ways of escaping these pressures. Unfortunately all of these habits have a negative impact on

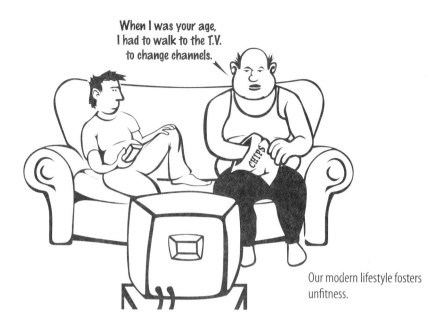

Our modern lifestyle fosters unfitness.

our physiological systems and affect our state of health. Thus, more than at any time in history, we need to seek out stimulating exercise.

Many men and women feel that their daily activities provide them with enough exercise for fitness. Running up and down stairs or standing all day at a job seems to be physical exertion. It is exertion, of course, but such limited activities do not use the lungs fully or stimulate the heart adequately. If normal, day-to-day activities leave you fatigued at the end of the day, then you need the increased energy and vitality that come from regular physical exertion. In other words, regular stimulation of the total body through vigorous exercise produces increased strength and endurance, characteristics associated with good health. These attributes cannot be acquired sitting at a desk all day, watching sports on television, riding elevators, or snacking on burgers, fries, and shakes.

Now that inactivity has been recognized as a threat to physiological well-being, some authorities suggest that exercise may be the cheapest preventive medicine in the world. Researchers in medicine, nutrition, psychology, physiology, and physical education agree that exercise, properly performed, is necessary for maintaining functional physical fitness. No responsible health educator would ever suggest that exercise is a panacea. But it is clear that, just as we need food, rest, and sleep, we need daily regular exercise to maintain our physical capacities. Physical fitness is not an end in itself, but a means to an

WAY OF LIFE
Detriments to Good Health

• Inactivity	• Poor management of stress
• Improper nutrition	• Excessive use of alcohol
• Smoking	• Drug abuse

end. It provides the basis for optimal physiological health and gives us the capacity to enjoy life to the fullest.

What Is Physical Fitness?

Most authors define physical fitness as the capacity to carry out everyday activities (work and play) without excessive fatigue and with enough reserve energy to deal with emergencies. Emphatically this definition is inadequate given our modern way of life. By such a definition, almost anyone can be classified as physically fit. The typical banker, merchant, nurse, or student can probably hustle to catch a bus, run up a flight of stairs to get to a meeting, or play in a weekend softball game. Nevertheless such a definition is not acceptable when we consider recent medical literature concerning the deleterious effects of inactivity on our health and well-being.

Inactivity—A Major Health Problem

Inactivity has been identified as a primary risk factor for coronary heart disease and related cardiovascular diseases. According to the American Heart Association, the United States has one of the highest death rates from cardiovascular disease in the world. Autopsy studies comparing people from highly affluent nations with those in less developed countries have led many medical authorities to suspect that diet, levels of physical activity, and other lifestyle habits common to Western society contribute to increased risk of diseases of the heart and blood vessels.

In addition, the modern man or woman does not live at an optimal fitness level. Most are satisfied simply to make minimal exertions. Physiological studies throughout the United States repeatedly bear out this conclusion. Longitudinal studies have shown a decline in physical fitness with age, but they also show that this trend can be changed by regular fitness training three to five days per week. This lack of optimal fitness is the result of our inactive lifestyle, which tends to make us sluggish and lazy. In addition, consuming foods high in cholesterol, fat, and sugar contributes to the decline in health and fitness. In many cases, such eating habits result in too many calories, which turn into unwanted ripples of fat. However, participating in a regular physical fitness program, properly planned and carried out, can help overcome the harmful health effects of living in a highly mechanized and computerized society. You probably do not need a high level of physical fitness to work in a world dominated by technical innovations, but regular physical activity is a necessity to maintain a healthy body.

Physical Fitness Defined

Physical fitness is the capability of the heart, blood vessels, lungs, and muscles to function at optimal efficiency. Optimal efficiency means the level of health needed for enthusiastic participation in daily tasks and recreational activities. Optimal physical fitness makes possible a lifestyle that the unfit cannot enjoy. To develop and maintain physical fitness requires vigorous effort by the total body. As you will learn later in this book, you do have to huff and puff a little. However, this does not mean punishing, exhausting exercise; it means working out within your capabilities. You will realize that the results are well worth the exertion and sweat required.

People who are physically fit look better, feel better, and possess the good health necessary for a happy and full life. The possession of optimal strength, muscle tone, and endurance, not only for emergencies but for everyday living, is the key to dynamic health.

Components of Physical Fitness

Strength, muscular endurance, flexibility, cardiorespiratory endurance, and body composition are the basic health-related components of physical fitness. These five characteristics are required for the healthy functioning of the body. Another trait, athletic skill, or motor ability, is often cited as a sixth fitness component. Although athletic skill is related to the other aspects of fitness, our main concern is with the health-related components. A rating of "good" in all of these areas indicates an acceptable level of physical fitness. Chapter 3 will assist you in determining your present fitness status. For now, we will briefly define each component to clarify its role in physical fitness.

Muscular Strength

Muscular strength, probably the most familiar component of fitness, is the maximal amount of force that can be generated by a muscle or group of muscles. It is typically assessed by determining how much weight a person can lift

> **WAY OF LIFE**
> **Components of Physical Fitness**
>
> - Muscular strength
> - Muscular endurance
> - Flexibility
>
> - Cardiorespiratory endurance
> - Body composition
> - Athletic skill/motor ability

only one time. Resistance training, or more specifically, strength training, is the mode of exercise used to increase muscle strength and to enlarge the muscles (that is, muscle hypertrophy).

Strength is fundamental in all sports. A lack of reasonable strength obviously contributes to poor performance in sports. Strength often seems to be lacking in the upper arms and shoulder region, especially in women. This lack of strength directly impairs one's ability to swing a golf club, to strike a tennis ball, or to carry out basic daily tasks.

Properly conducted resistance training programs, such as working with barbells, are the most efficient means for gaining strength. Such training may also result in increased muscle mass. In Chapter 7, we discuss resistance training techniques for the development of strength.

Muscular Endurance

This trait is often used synonymously, but incorrectly, with strength. **Muscular endurance** is the capacity of a muscle to contract repeatedly over a period of time. Also, it refers to the ability of the muscle to hold a fixed, or static, contraction. In other words, it is the ability to apply strength and sustain it. Your ability to perform as many pull-ups as possible or to hold a bent-arm hang is an indication of your muscular endurance. The capacity of your legs to perform in an endurance race, your arm to repeatedly swing a tennis racquet, or your hands to grip a golf club firmly throughout a round of golf are also examples of muscular endurance. Even activities around the home, such as shoveling snow, washing windows, painting, and cleaning, all require some degree of prolonged muscular exertion.

Flexibility

Flexibility is the ability to move the joints—to bend, stretch, and twist. Maintenance of good joint mobility can decrease the risk for muscle injury and soreness, while inflexible joints and muscles increase the risk. The need for flexibility varies with your specific needs. In swimming, shoulder and ankle flexibility is important for efficient movement through the water. In the martial arts, the muscles of the legs, arms, and abdomen need a full range of movement. Even walking and jogging, seemingly effortless movements, require some degree of flexibility in the major muscle groups.

Cardiorespiratory Endurance

Although the physical fitness components discussed previously are important, **cardiorespiratory endurance** is the most essential physical fitness component. Your very life depends on the capacity of your heart, blood vessels, and lungs to deliver nutrients and oxygen to your tissues and to remove wastes. Efficient functioning of the heart and lungs is required for optimal enjoyment of activities such as running, swimming, and cycling. Most important, good cardiorespiratory endurance helps you maintain vigorous everyday living.

Body Composition

Recently **body composition** has been included as one of the components of physical fitness. This component refers to the relative amounts of fat and lean body tissue (such as muscle and bone) that make up your body. Equations have been developed for estimating one's relative body fat.

Relative body fat is the percentage of total body weight that is fat. Carrying extra body fat not only affects physical functioning but also is associated with

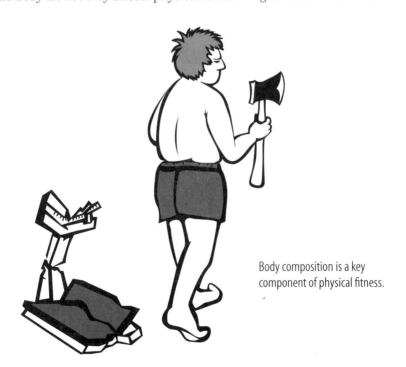

Body composition is a key
component of physical fitness.

poor health and physical fitness. Research evidence strongly suggests that physical inactivity is a principal cause of excess weight gain, especially in the form of fat. And obesity certainly increases one's risk for serious medical problems.

Regular exercise is a positive approach to weight control. In fact, fit people burn more fat calories than do the unfit, because of their enhanced ability to utilize fats for energy during exercise and their favorable body composition. In other words, fit individuals possess a higher percentage of muscle, which is "hungry" tissue requiring more energy than fat tissue. Basically the fit person at rest burns more calories than the less fit, thus decreasing the risk for fat gain. How fat are you? What is your desired weight? Methods for answering these questions are presented in Chapter 3. Also, in Chapter 10, you will find updated information on the role of exercise and nutrition in maintaining your proper body weight.

Athletic Skill

The ability of the nerves to receive and provide impulses that result in smooth, coordinated muscular movements is a wonder of the human body. It is evident in the flawless performances of elite figure skaters and other great athletes. Although a desirable attribute, having a high degree of **athletic skill,** or motor ability, is not essential for maintaining a good level of physical health. Your ability to dodge, to control your balance, to react and move quickly—that is, to have your muscles function harmoniously and efficiently—reflects your general athletic skill. Athletic skill can usually be evaluated with simple tests. Such tests as the vertical jump (requiring explosive power), agility run (requiring speed, balance, and agility), and 20-yard dash (requiring speed of body movement) have traditionally been used as measures of motor skill and general athletic ability. Tests of this type have always been popular with the athletically inclined.

Fundamental Reasons for Physical Fitness

You might ask, why do I need cardiorespiratory endurance? or, why do I need an increase in strength? The answer is simple: It is foolish to live at your minimal potential. You need to have more than the minimal capacity for exertion to carry out everyday activities efficiently, let alone to deal with emergencies. Optimally functioning cardiorespiratory and muscular systems enable you to do so, and physical fitness leads to optimal performance of both. In addition, and most important, physical fitness enhances your capacity to enjoy life fully. Throughout this book, we will explain how a good fitness program improves cardiorespiratory and muscular functioning.

Optimal Muscular and Cardiorespiratory Health

It is a physiological fact that the human body needs stimulating exercise. When your total body is subjected to regular physical activity, requiring a vigorous stress on the heart, lungs, and muscles, your physiological functions improve. For example, the fit person adjusts to increased physical demands and returns to a normal state more quickly than the unfit person. At rest, a physically fit heart beats at a lower rate and pumps more blood per beat. As the result of regular exercise, an individual's capacity to use oxygen increases substantially, thereby enabling that person to perform more physical work. Although regular exercise is not a cure-all, it is a sound means for maintaining a high level of health. There is no scientific evidence showing harmful effects from regular exercise in a healthy person. But an abundance of research now strongly supports the theory that regular, vigorous exercise helps keep healthy hearts healthy and may prevent heart disease.

A Full Life

People who keep fit live greatly fuller lives. They can do a day's work with ease; they can meet most emergencies; and they can extend their recreational activities to a second set of tennis, an extra nine holes of golf, or an extra mile of hiking.

Today more and more people are becoming interested in recreation and sports. Activities such as backpacking, roller-blading, cross-country skiing, scuba diving, and mountain biking are increasingly popular. However, for complete enjoyment, participation in these activities requires a level of physical fitness beyond that needed in everyday life. To be pleasurable, a hike up a mountain or a scuba dive in a lake requires adequate physical conditioning. In other words, to enjoy your recreational endeavors fully, you need to be in shape.

Being physically fit provides the robust health and the excess energy needed to fully enjoy life. Simply put, it means doing more and doing it better. We don't necessarily exercise simply to prevent heart disease, to live longer, or to shed excess fat. Rather, we exercise to arrive at an increased physical capacity that allows us to enjoy a full life. Being able to do more things competently and enjoyably makes for healthier, happier lives.

Summary

Your body was made to be used. Unfortunately, in today's fast-paced world, your body cannot always handle the stress of daily activities. Our highly mechanized and computerized society has changed the way we live. Physical work and labor have been minimized in carrying out daily living. The proliferation of all kinds of remote, automated, and innovative technical devices has diminished the need for physical exertion.

Since ancient times, we have known that the body needs regular exercise. Active people tend to be healthier. Although not a guarantee of health, regular exercise more and more is viewed as the key to health and wellness. Exercise can be the "positive do" in your life. Do exercise!

Throughout this book, we suggest ways to help you develop better physical conditioning and, hopefully, better health. Life is a menu of choices. You must act and move ahead with the suggestion to exercise. No one can do it for you. There is no pill you can take to make you physically fit. Good luck!

Key Words

ATHLETIC SKILL/MOTOR ABILITY: The ability of muscles to function harmoniously and efficiently, resulting in smooth, coordinated muscular movement; a reflection of general athletic ability.

BODY COMPOSITION: The relative amounts of fat and lean body tissue (such as muscle and bone) that make up one's body.

CARDIORESPIRATORY ENDURANCE: The capacity of the heart, blood vessels, and lungs to function efficiently during vigorous, sustained activity such as running, swimming, or cycling.

FLEXIBILITY: The range of movement of a specific joint and its corresponding muscle groups.

HEALTH: The general condition of one's physical, intellectual, social, emotional, and spiritual being. Health is best depicted as a continuum with death and wellness at its extremes.

MUSCULAR ENDURANCE: The capacity of a muscle to contract repeatedly or to hold a fixed or static contraction over a period of time.

MUSCULAR STRENGTH: The maximal amount of force generated by a muscle or group of muscles.

PHYSICAL FITNESS: A physiological state blending health-related and skill-related components that reflects the body's ability to meet physical challenges and resist diseases associated with sedentary living.

WELLNESS: The state of health that results when physical, intellectual, spiritual, social, and emotional components are all at optimal levels.

A Way of Life Library

Dickman, S. R. *Pathways to Wellness.* Champaign, IL: Human Kinetics, 1988.

Haskell W. L. J. B. Wolffe Memorial Lecture: "Health Consequences of Physical Activity: Understanding and Challenges Regarding Dose-Response." *Medicine & Science in Sports & Exercise* 26 (1994): 649–60.

Powers, S. K., and S. L. Dodd. *Total Fitness: Exercise, Nutrition, and Wellness.* Boston: Allyn & Bacon, 1996.

Williams, M. *Lifetime Fitness and Wellness.* Dubuque, IA: Wm. C. Brown, 1996.

CHAPTER 2

Getting Started and Staying with It

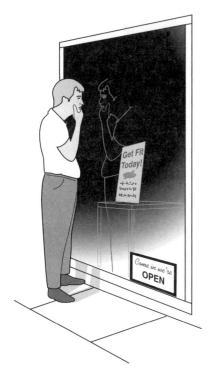

The key to making physical fitness a way of life is to assume responsibility for your own workouts. In the long run (no pun intended), you are accountable only to yourself in practicing and maintaining a healthy, active lifestyle. Any knowledge, direction, or encouragement gained from this book can only serve as a catalyst to a lifetime of dynamic physical health. If you continue to exercise vigorously on a regular basis, you will gradually change in a variety of ways. These training effects manifest themselves in improved functioning of your heart, lungs, and muscles, both at rest and during physical exertion.

The following chapters discuss the benefits of each type of training in more depth. In reality, these physiological benefits may simply be a bonus. Perhaps the positive feelings and mental highs experienced by many fitness enthusiasts are the true benefits of exercise. Regardless, you will experience none of these benefits if you do not turn your knowledge into action. This chapter may increase your motivation as it discusses the psychological benefits derived from exercise. It also gives concrete suggestions for making your workouts an enjoyable priority in your life.

As you read this chapter, keep these statements in mind:

- Exercise can have positive effects on the mind as well as the body.

- There is no magical or easy way to get or keep in shape; it does take physical effort performed over a lifetime.
- Maintaining optimal fitness can be a struggle at times.
- Coping with the weather, the limited availability of facilities, the lack of time, physical problems, and just plain laziness are some of the stumbling blocks we all face.
- Keeping your commitment to regular exercise involves overcoming obstacles and balancing priorities.

The evidence is conclusive that exercise has positive physiological effects on the body. The psychological benefits of exercise are more difficult to assess objectively. However, the number of people who testify to such benefits is impressive. And some research suggests that regular participation in fitness activities is associated with an overall feeling of well-being. Although this may be difficult for the nonexerciser to accept, most physical fitness advocates feel there is a definite relationship among physical, intellectual, social, emotional, and spiritual well-being.

Being fit bolsters your self-image and helps you to be more positive about yourself and those around you. Studies indicate that regular exercisers are less tired, are more relaxed, have higher self-esteem, and are more productive at work. Dr. Kenneth Cooper of the famed Cooper Aerobics Center in Dallas believes strongly that people who are physically fit tend to be psychologically fit as well. They exhibit a "fitness glow"—they feel better, look better, and have an improved self-image.

Exercise provides a diversion from everyday tasks and relaxes the mind. The late George Sheehan, cardiologist, runner, and author of several best-selling books on running, asserted that it is the psychology rather than the physiology

WAY OF LIFE
Mind Matters

- Regular exercise can be physically and psychologically uplifting.
- An exercise-induced "high" is very individual and may not be experienced by all active people.

- Workouts should be seen as a chance to "play."
- Feeling better, looking better, and improving your self-esteem collectively contribute to your "fitness glow."

of fitness that is important. He used the words *play* and *exercise* interchangeably in his writings. According to Sheehan, "Play provides . . . physical grace, psychological ease, and personal integrity. . . . One who plays is fulfilling himself and becoming the person he is." He believed that "exercise must be play or it will do little good." Although his words refer mainly to running, any fitness activity can become play, provide a feeling of exhilaration, and refresh the soul. People who exercise regularly simply feel—and act—more alive.

Research also suggests that exercise can be an antidepressant. Physicians have had remarkable results treating depressed patients with exercise. Some patients have abandoned medications, reduced or eliminated smoking and drinking, changed other unhealthy habits, and improved their overall well-being with exercise.

Strategies for a Lifetime of Physical Activity

Despite its many benefits, you may still have doubts as to whether exercise is for you. Perhaps you have developed some negative attitudes from past experiences: "Exercise is painful," or "I've never been good in physical activities," or "Running isn't for a clod like me." Negative attitudes caused by unpleasant memories need to be overcome. Often these unpleasant memories reinforce the fear that you can't succeed at an exercise program. Self-doubt can be debilitating, but we all experience it at some point in our lives, and we can overcome it. The good news is that the exercise guidelines presented in this book can lead virtually everyone, regardless of past experiences, to experience a successful lifetime of physical activity.

Most likely you are reading this book in conjunction with a class in which the why and how of healthy exercise are emphasized. This section will provide some tips on how you can assume responsibility for your own health and well-being both presently and long after the class ends. Your instructor can help and encourage you in the early stages of your program, but the ultimate commitment to regular training rests with you. Keeping physically fit will always take effort. But we hope you will reach the point at which you will be working out not because you have to, but because you want to.

Making and Keeping the Commitment

Do you accept that exercising on a regular basis is a desirable behavior? If so, the next step involves prioritizing your daily activities to achieve this desirable behavior. *It is time not only to think fitness and health but to practice fitness and health.* Whatever your reason for starting an exercise program, you must pledge to stay with it. If you can keep your commitment during the early weeks of

- Lack of time
- Lack of facilities
- Lack of knowledge
- Lack of success
- Lack of family or peer support

- Illness (your own and others')
- Family obligations
- Procrastination
- Bad weather
- Injuries

your program, you will be well on your way to a lifetime of enjoyable and beneficial activity. In fact, you will have passed the first dropout hump. As a general rule, it takes at least three to four months for most people to fully appreciate the pleasures of stimulating exercise. Statistics show that long-term **exercise adherence,** which is the practice of closely following an exercise program, increases significantly after one year of regular exercising. Therefore

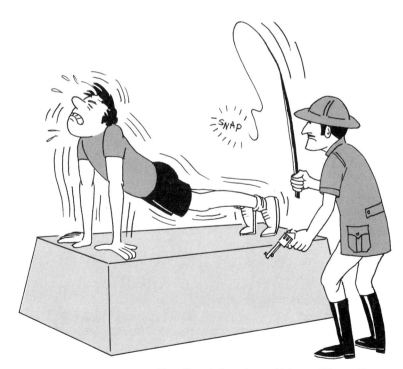

You will reach the point at which you will be working out not because you have to, but because you want to.

you must stay with it long enough to fully realize the rewards. When you reach this point, you will probably be working out because you want to.

Living at optimal physiological health should be a top priority, warranting the investment of a reasonable amount of time and effort. There are 168 hours in a week. All you need is about four 30-minute workouts of sustained exercise per week to attain and maintain a reasonable fitness level. That's only 2 hours a week! Throw in a couple more hours for warm-ups and cool-downs, showers, and so on, and you still have over 160 hours at your disposal—a small investment of time and effort for such a large and beneficial return.

Getting Started

Keep two things in mind as you move on to the next chapters. First, you can never begin too low on the exercise charts, and the steps you take can never be too small. In other words, proceed carefully and don't be in a hurry. Injuries and discouragement can result when you try to do too much too soon.

Expect to feel "effort" when you exercise. Even a bit of discomfort is not unusual when you start out. This feeling will vary from day to day and from person to person. The important point to remember is that *if you are quite uncomfortable or fatigued an hour or more after a workout, you are probably overdoing it.* Therefore you need to make some adjustment in your next workout. The chapters to follow will show you how to keep your workouts reasonably comfortable and how to avoid unnecessary fatigue.

Second, don't try to change everything at once. A regular exercise program may provide an incentive to change such negative habits as smoking and overeating. But first, start getting into shape. Then you can more effectively tackle the problems of smoking and controlling your weight. Embarking on an exercise program while cutting down on cigarettes and maintaining a strict, low-calorie diet is usually inviting failure. It takes an unusual person to make all these adjustments at once. So take it one step at a time. Begin by making activity and physical fitness a high priority and becoming active. As you progress and your body becomes more attuned to exercise, then consider making gradual changes in smoking and eating habits.

Staying with It

If you are in a regularly scheduled class, staying with an exercise program is generally not too difficult. However, once you have completed the class, you may confront stumbling blocks. Lack of time, illness (your own and others'), family obligations, procrastination (we all experience this), bad weather, and various types of injuries, to name just a few obstacles, can easily sidetrack a well-intentioned fitness endeavor. Such setbacks can be disconcerting and, for

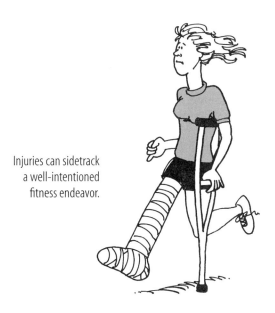

Injuries can sidetrack
a well-intentioned
fitness endeavor.

some people, reason enough to quit. Keep in mind that you should not become overly concerned if you absolutely cannot participate in your regular program on a given day. Even with the best plans and intentions, an occasional break in your fitness routine is inevitable. Just because you miss a workout, all is not lost! Rather than be unreasonably hard on yourself, simply accept your day off and get back on track. Adopting the attitude that fitness is for life will put a missed workout in healthy perspective. Following are some strategies to overcoming typical obstacles.

Establish Fitness Priorities

When confronted with the question "What do you want to get from your exercise program?" many people state that they want to "get in shape." This phrase means different things to different people. For some, getting in shape means decreasing body fat; for others, it means improving cardiorespiratory endurance. By familiarizing yourself with the various physical fitness components (see Chapter 1), you can identify and prioritize your fitness goals. No one training mode will simultaneously cause optimal improvements in all fitness components. Thus it is important to prioritize which fitness components you currently want to work on most. This will help you establish your fitness goals. For example, if your current goal is to lower body fat, then perform aerobic exercises that burn the most calories. An exercise program designed with fitness priorities in mind will ensure positive results and further motivate making fitness a way of life.

Set Some Goals

The rewards of exercise become especially clear when you set specific goals and then work to reach those goals. For example, perhaps after your 1.5-mile run test (see Chapter 3) you realize that you need to improve your cardiorespiratory endurance. Let's say you wish to bring a 14-minute time down to 12 minutes. Once you have set this specific goal, use the suggestions in the following chapters to design a program that allows you to reach your goal in a reasonable time frame. In subsequent chapters, you'll learn how often, how long, and how hard to perform various exercises to reach your goals.

Follow a Plan

A well-planned workout enhances your chances for improvement. However, do not expect to see instant improvement or expect each workout to result in progress. Gains in physical fitness come in spurts. Every day will not be a glorious one, and each session will not leave you euphoric, but you should feel good after each workout. The progressive workout tables in Chapters 5 and 6 will help you through good days and bad days. Each step on these charts is designed so that you can complete it without becoming overly fatigued and still receive the necessary stimulation to your heart, lungs, and muscles. Eventually you will not need the charts, but you will need to plan your workouts so you can maintain your fitness. Planning a program is relatively easy. However, carrying it out on a regular basis is the challenge.

Find a Time

Finding time is the most difficult problem for many people. But time isn't hard to find if you know where to look for it and have made exercise a priority in your life. You need to honestly appraise your schedule and accept that some sacrifices may be necessary. For example, early morning may be the best time for your workouts because there are fewer conflicts and interruptions at that time of day. Take a good look at your day's activities and find the time that best suits your schedule. Many people unwind from a stressful day by exercising in the late afternoon.

Find a Place to Work Out

The best place to work out is where you like it most! Keep in mind that this location may change over time as you improve your fitness levels, change your goals, or add new activities. Most forms of cardiorespiratory exercise can be enjoyed both outdoors and indoors, with other exercisers or alone, using complex equipment or nothing more than a good pair of shoes. Finding a place to work out can be as easy as stepping out your front door or walking down the hall to your company's fitness center or strolling to your campus's athletic complex. Some key attractions to a workout spot include convenience, safety, motivation, and variety. This is why many people choose to exercise at home or in their own neighborhood. Measuring workout distances can be as easy as checking your car odometer before and after driving your running or biking route. If possible, pick at least two (and preferably more) different routes so that you can vary your scenery daily. If one route includes hills, map out another more level one for alternate days. From a crime prevention standpoint, you are safer if your route (and even time of day) is not predictable and does not follow a pattern.

If you enjoy the camaraderie of fellow exercisers, need professional advice and guidance for your workouts, or frequently switch activities and enjoy a variety of equipment choices, a commercial fitness center membership may be your best option. When choosing a commercial fitness center, look for a location within a short drive or walk from home or work. Request a "try before you buy" membership or at least a guest pass to make certain the staff, equipment, and classes are worth your investment. Ask current members questions to obtain unbiased information. Refer to the American College of Sports Medicine's *Health/Fitness Facility Consumer Selection Guide* (see A Way of Life Library). Although currently there are no nationwide certifications or standards of quality that fitness centers must legally adhere to, consumers can inquire whether a center meets the American College of Sports Medicine's standards and guidelines (see A Way of Life Library). Adherence to the guidelines at least suggests that a facility recognizes the basics in quality and safety.

If possible, choose a specific time for your regular workout. Experience has shown that setting aside a specific time of day to exercise will increase your chances of working out on a regular basis. Occasionally, because of other obligations, you might have to be flexible and change the time of your workout. However, setting aside a specific time for exercise lessens the chance that you will put it off. It's easy to say, "I'll do it tonight," and then when evening comes say, "I'll do it in the morning." Choose a definite time that's best for you, and stick to it.

Make It Social

Another tactic to keep you on a regular schedule is to work out with a friend, roommate, or perhaps spouse. Meeting someone or picking someone up and driving to an exercise area together works for many people. Working out with friends can provide an incentive to keep you going.

Have the Right Equipment and Clothing

For serious fitness workouts, street clothes are usually too confining for efficient and enjoyable movement. Today clothing specifically designed to maximize comfort and mobility is readily available. Perhaps a special outfit is not necessary to begin your fitness training, but you will quickly discover that garments like tight-fitting shorts or jeans can hinder movement or be too warm. Fitnesswear is lightweight, streamlined, unrestricting, durable, and often protective. Gone are the days of the "sauna suit"—rubberized pants and tops that caused exercisers to sweat excessively. Although people could, in fact, lose weight wearing the suits, the weight lost was mostly water, not fat. Once exercisers drank water, they regained the weight. More important, these suits do not allow sweat evaporation, which can lead to dangerous overheating of the body. Your best option is to wear clothing that allows your body to cool itself in the most effective way possible.

If you choose to exercise outdoors during the dark hours, you would be wise to incorporate reflective items into your fitness wardrobe. Lightweight reflective vests and reflective tape placed strategically on the back of shoes and gloves make you much more visible to motorists sharing your streets. Small blinking lights can also be worn around your ankle or upper arm to enhance your visibility from a distance. In case of emergency, it is a good idea to carry some sort of identification with your name and phone number. You can purchase special tags and bracelets at sporting goods stores. Alternatively you can simply record the information with indelible ink on the outside borders of your shoes.

Drinking water before, during, and after any form of exercise is a must. Lightweight plastic water bottles have been commonplace on bikes for years, but now bottle holders are available for virtually all cardiorespiratory exercise equipment. Even fitness walkers can wear specially designed belts with "holsters" for one or more water bottles. Cross-country skiers can also wear canteenlike containers sewn into hip belts. However, because the water can be cold against a skier's lower back, thick material such as a small towel can be placed between the hips and the belt. Swimmers, too, should be encouraged to fill a water bottle and leave it on the pool deck at the end of the lane for frequent gulps.

As you will learn in Chapter 4, exercise intensity is an important variable in correctly designing a workout. Checking your pulse at least once fairly early in your exercise session can assure you that you are achieving a cardiorespiratory training effect. Some people prefer electronic gadgets, such as a pulse monitor. Pulse monitors typically include electrodes and a transmitter worn around the rib cage on a belt. The electrodes pick up your pulse and transmit it to a receiver that resembles a wristwatch. The receiver can be programmed to beep when you drop below or exceed your target heart-rate range. Some models can even be downloaded onto your computer for a display of your exercise heart rates taken at different intervals throughout your workout.

For many people, exercise is the highlight of their day, and performing the repetitive motions of cardiorespiratory activities frees their minds to think creatively. However, some individuals enjoy exercise more if they incorporate

- Establish fitness priorities.
- Set some goals.
- Follow a plan.
- Find a time.
- Find a place.
- Make it social.
- Have the right equipment and clothing.
- Keep a record.
- Add variety.

reading or listening to music or watching television at the same time. For outdoor activities, lightweight radio headsets can be worn like a headband, while portable cassette tape and compact disc players can be carried in small pouches slung low on the hips. Just make certain to maintain a volume that allows you to easily hear vehicles (and dogs!) quite a distance before they reach you. Indoor exercise in front of the television lets exercisers catch up on news and favorite programs. Book and magazine racks can easily be mounted on equipment frames. However, one point to stress with all of these diversions is the importance of maintaining intensity, form, and safety at all times.

Keep a Record

Motivation is increased when you keep a record of your workouts. This allows you to track your fitness program. Such a record is most helpful during the early weeks of training. It actually becomes fun to note items such as your activity, the duration of the workout, the distance covered if you swam or ran or cycled, and your feelings after the workout. A special exercise log, or even a calendar, works especially well.

Add Variety

The old adage "variety is the spice of life" holds true for exercise. Many people tend to perform the same exercise program day in and day out. Because exercise is for life, doing the same thing can be downright boring. Don't be afraid to try new exercise activities! Furthermore, no single program will meet your fitness needs as you go through life. Your fitness goals will change periodically, and you should adapt your program to achieve those new goals. The more you learn about exercise, the more comfortable you will become at making changes to your program. In fact, many fitness enthusiasts regularly participate in a variety of activities such as biking on one day, running another, and swimming another, in a practice known as **cross-training.** You can also add variety by changing training location, time of day, and exercise partners. Your life is full of variety, so why shouldn't your exercise program be as well?

Summary

Let's be honest—staying fit will always take effort. But the rewards are well worth that effort. As your fitness level improves, you form habits that become part of your daily routine throughout life. And as you adjust to a more physical lifestyle, you will increasingly enjoy the full benefits of exercise. It can be done if you make an effort to stay with your regular workouts.

If you stick with your program for at least three or four months, you will be over the first dropout hump. Statistics show that long-term adherence rates increase significantly after one year of regular exercising. So what does it take to get beyond these first few dropout points? It takes a sincere commitment on your part along with a plan that can work for you. You need to set goals that you can realistically achieve. Becoming fit happens not in one big leap, but in small, steady steps. Develop your plan, keep a record, work out with friends, and periodically evaluate your progress. Consider your time, effort, and devotion to regular workouts as a major investment in yourself. If you miss a workout or get ill and need to rest, do not feel guilty. Simply get back to your program as soon as possible. Making physical fitness a way of life gives you a feeling of accomplishment and the ability to do more things with a sense of energy. Living life to the fullest is fun!

Key Words

CROSS-TRAINING: A training practice in which a variety of different exercise activities are used to accomplish fitness goals.

EXERCISE ADHERENCE: The practice of closely following a regular exercise program.

A Way of Life Library

American College of Sports Medicine. *ACSM Fitness Book.* Champaign, IL: Human Kinetics, 1992.

American College of Sports Medicine. *ACSM's Health/Fitness Facility Standards and Guidelines.* Champaign, IL: Human Kinetics, 1992.

American College of Sports Medicine. *ACSM's Health/Fitness Facility Consumer Selection Guide.* 317-637-9200, ext. 127.

Cooper, K. H. *The Aerobics Program for Total Well-Being.* Toronto: Bantam Books, 1982.

Franks, B. D., and E. T. Howley. *Fitness Facts.* Champaign, IL: Human Kinetics, 1989.

Sheehan, G. *Dr. Sheehan on Running.* Mountain View, CA: World Publications, 1975.

CHAPTER 3

Assessing Your Fitness

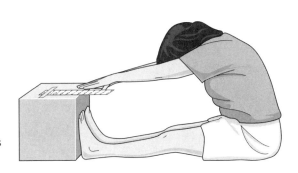

This chapter will assist
you in evaluating your
present physical fitness
status to identify your
strengths and weak-
nesses. This evaluation will provide the basis for setting up an exercise
program that is safe, reasonable, and effective. Also, it will enable you to
determine the effectiveness of your individualized exercise program.

The tests included in this chapter primarily measure the health-
related components of physical fitness, as well as some skill-related
components. The tests are easy to administer and cover the major areas
of fitness evaluation: body composition, flexibility, motor skill, muscular
strength, cardiorespiratory endurance, and muscular endurance.
Although physical fitness tests have limitations, these tests will provide
you with a rough estimate of your physical fitness status. Not only will
you gain insight into the fitness of your muscles, heart, lungs, and circulatory system, but you will discover through an assessment of your body
fat what is a reasonable weight for you.

As you read this chapter, keep these statements in mind:

- Testing should not dominate your exercise program. Physical fitness measurements, however, will not only help you in evaluating your present condition but assist you in setting reasonable goals.
- The intent of self-testing is to help you evaluate your present level of physical fitness and, later on, the effectiveness of your program.
- For men age 45 or over, women age 55 or over, and anyone who has not
  recently been active, a medical exam is recommended before attempting
  these tests.

- In order to obtain an all-inclusive evaluation, tests representing traits for each of the health-related physical fitness components should be utilized.
- Scale weight gives no indication as to a person's body fat. Only body composition determination methods can indicate if you have too much body fat.

Physical fitness means more than bulging muscles or a trim waistline. A lean appearance, although desirable, does not necessarily reflect your physical fitness. No matter how you look, or even how strong you are, you have a low level of fitness if your heart is unable to meet the circulatory demands of prolonged work. Many men and women, for instance, appear very fit but tire easily while carrying out their everyday activities.

Each individual is unique, with different abilities in various physical and mental tasks. In addition, all people have their own physiological limitations. This chapter will help you develop a practical testing program for appraising your fitness so that you can set up a program that is appropriate for you.

It is only human to be curious about how you compare with others. Although physical fitness measurements afford you this opportunity, it is more important to use your data to help set up a reasonable program that meets your needs. Later on, you will want to repeat these tests to assess the effectiveness of your training program.

Physical fitness testing should not dominate a conditioning program. However, if used properly, your test results can serve as a highly effective motivational device. The classification charts presented in this chapter for the various tests can show your strengths and weaknesses. Comparing your test results with the charts will give you insight into your physical capabilities. In addition, it will help you evaluate the effectiveness of your training program, whether it involves running, swimming, weight training, or a combination of activities. Consequently don't be overly concerned with what other people can or cannot do. The self-tests in this chapter will help you make your own before-and-after comparisons. Fitness is individual, so measure your own improvement and

WAY OF LIFE
Reasons for Fitness Testing

- To establish one's fitness status
- To evaluate the effectiveness of a training program
- To use as a basis for setting goals
- To use results to plan proper workouts
- To provide motivation for starting and adhering to an exercise program

watch your own progress. By following the testing procedures carefully, you can find out whether you need to improve any or all of the components of physical fitness.

Finally, if you are in doubt about your state of health, check with your physician before attempting any of these vigorous tests. This is very important for persons over 30, especially for anyone who has not recently been physically active.

Physical Fitness Test Battery

The tests in this chapter have all been used successfully in recent years to measure the basic components of physical fitness. They were selected because they provide for uniformity in scoring, consistency in measuring, and overall ease in administering. Also, minimal time and equipment are required to perform these tests. In some cases, you may have access to more extensive tests to evaluate your fitness. Regardless of what set of tests you use, going through a **test battery**—a series of tests used to measure the various components of physical fitness—can help you establish a fitness baseline.

The tests are grouped into the following areas: (1) body composition, (2) flexibility, (3) athletic skill performance, (4) muscular strength, (5) muscular endurance, and (6) cardiorespiratory endurance. Reasonably high scores in all of these tests are necessary for you to be classified as physically fit. The rationale for the tests and the instructions for carrying them out are presented in the sections that follow. For your convenience, we have included a data sheet on which to record your test measures (see Figure 3.1a and b).

Following is a suggested order of testing. For best results, take two days to perform the tests. Make sure to follow the same order for the tests during both the initial testing and any follow-up testing. Also, note the length of rest periods between tests, and use the same rest periods when performing follow-up testing.

Suggested Order of Testing

- Day 1:
    Body Composition
    Flexibility: Trunk Flexion
    Motor Skill: Vertical Jump
    Motor Skill: 20-Yard Dash
    Motor Skill: Agility Run
    Muscular Strength: Chest Press
    Muscular Strength: Leg Press

FIGURE 3.1A
Fitness Assessment Data Sheet: Day 1

Name: _____ Date: _____

Age: _____ Height: _____ Weight: _____

Body Composition (skinfold measures in millimeters)

	Measure 1	Measure 2	Measure 3	Average of 3 Measures
Triceps	_____	_____	_____	_____
Subscapula	_____	_____	_____	_____
Midaxillary	_____	_____	_____	_____
Suprailiac	_____	_____	_____	_____
Abdomen	_____	_____	_____	_____
Thigh	_____	_____	_____	_____

Sum of 6 averages = _____

Percent body fat (see Figure 3.3) _____

Norm category _____

Trunk Flexion (in inches)

Measure 1 _____ Measure 2 _____ Measure 3 _____ Best of 3 _____

Norm category _____

Vertical Jump (to nearest ½ inch)

Standing reach _____

Jump 1 _____ Jump 2 _____ Jump 3 _____ Best of 3 _____

Best of 3 minus standing reach _____ (vertical jump height)

Norm category _____

20-Yard Dash (to nearest 1/10 second)

Run 1 _____ Run 2 _____ Run 3 _____ Fastest of 3 _____

Norm category _____

Agility Run (to nearest 1/10 second)

Time _____ Norm category _____

Chest Press (in pounds)

Measure 1 _____ Measure 2 _____ Measure 3 _____ Best of 3 _____

Best measure divided by body weight _____ (1 RM/body weight)

Norm category _____

Leg Press (in pounds)

Measure 1 _____ Measure 2 _____ Measure 3 _____ Best of 3 _____

Best measure divided by body weight _____ (1 RM/body weight)

Norm category _____

FIGURE 3.1B
Fitness Assessment Data Sheet: Day 2

Push-ups (repetitions)
Number of push-ups in 1 minute _____ Norm category _____

Abdominal Crunches (repetitions)
Number of abdominal crunches in 1 minute _____ Norm category _____

1.5-Mile Run (in minutes:seconds)
Time for 1.5 mile run _____ Norm category _____

Step Test (heart rate)
Recovery heart rate 1:00 to 1:30 _____
Recovery heart rate 2:00 to 2:30 _____
Recovery heart rate 3:00 to 3:30 _____
Sum of 3 recovery heart rates (recovery index) _____
Norm category _____

- Day 2:

    Muscular Endurance: Push-ups

    Muscular Endurance: Abdominal Crunches

    Cardiorespiratory Endurance: 1.5-Mile Run or Step Test

In each section, you will also find tables that list test results for men and women and provide scales on which you can rate your own performance. Remember not to get carried away comparing your scores to the scores in the tables or the performance of others. If you score low in all tests or only in one or two, consider the reasons, and design your training program to do something about it.

Evaluating Body Composition

Weighing yourself on a scale tells you nothing about your body composition because it does not discriminate between **fat weight** and **lean body weight** (composed primarily of muscles and bones). Thus trying to track changes in body fat based on body weight can be misleading and frustrating. For example, certain types of exercise programs can increase lean body weight and decrease fat weight, resulting in little change in body weight even though fat was lost. The best way to track changes in body composition is through laboratory techniques such as underwater weighing or through skinfold measures. Underwater weighing is considered the "gold standard" for determination of body composition. However, it requires expensive equipment and a trained technician. Skinfold measures are determined using relatively inexpensive **skinfold calipers,** which measure the thickness of fat lying immediately below the surface of the skin. Unfortunately skinfold measurement is also best performed by experienced professionals. These services are offered through university, hospital, or fitness center health/wellness programs at a small cost (generally $5 to $35). If possible, *we highly recommend that you get your body composition measured prior to beginning your program.* For your information, we have included instructions on the proper technique for measuring skinfolds and the location of six sites commonly measured.

The skinfold measures can be used in two ways. One is to estimate your percent body fat. Another interesting way, one that can be less demoralizing for those who are self-conscious or don't want to know their body fat, is simply to use the sum of the skinfolds. Keeping track of changes in the sum of the skinfolds lets you know whether you are gaining or losing fat over time. Furthermore, it can give you an indication of where you are losing the most body fat.

The anatomical landmarks for the six skinfold sites are as follows (see Figure 3.2):

1. *Tricep:* A vertical fold on the back of the upper arm midway between the shoulder and elbow joints
2. *Subscapula:* A diagonal fold on the back immediately below the lower angle of the scapula
3. *Midaxillary:* A vertical fold on the side of the body (mid-armpit) at the level of the lower end of the sternum
4. *Suprailiac:* A diagonal fold on the side of the body (mid-armpit) just above the top of the hip bone (crest of the ilium)
5. *Abdomen:* A vertical fold on the abdomen approximately 2 centimeters (1 inch) to the side of the navel
6. *Thigh:* A vertical fold on the front of the thigh midway between the hip and knee joints

PROCEDURE: Skinfold measures are taken on the right side of your body (even for left-handed persons) while you are standing. At the appropriate site, grasp a fold of skin using the thumb and forefinger of your left hand. Most of the skinfolds taken at the different sites are vertical folds; the folds taken at the subscapular and suprailiac sites are diagonal. The diagonal folds are picked up on a slight slant that follows the natural folding of the skin. While holding the skinfold with your left thumb and index finger, place the caliper pinchers over the fold about a half inch below your fingers. (*Note:* It is important to maintain your hold on the fold with your left hand throughout the measuring process.) Release the spring lever on the calipers and, within 2 seconds, take the skinfold

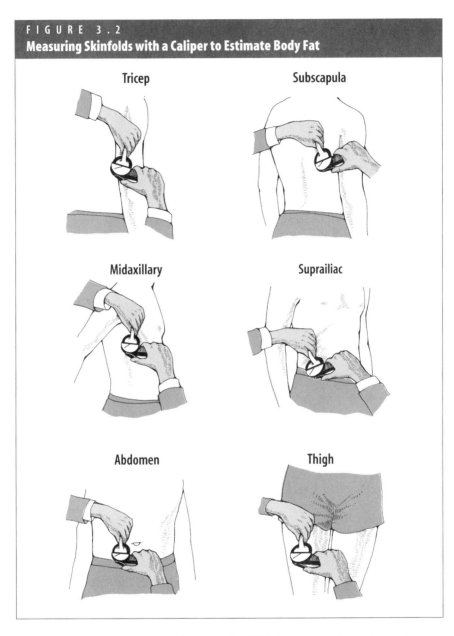

FIGURE 3.2
Measuring Skinfolds with a Caliper to Estimate Body Fat

Tricep

Subscapula

Midaxillary

Suprailiac

Abdomen

Thigh

measurement. Move to the next skinfold site. Rotate from site to site until you have taken three measures for each. Average the three measures for each site and then add the averages together to get your sum of the skinfold measures. To estimate percent body fat, use the nomogram (see Figure 3.3) and the designated sites in Figure 3.2. Table 3.1 gives the norms for body composition.

FIGURE 3.3A

Nomograms for Conversion of Skinfolds to Body Density[1] and Percent Body Fat[2] (Women)

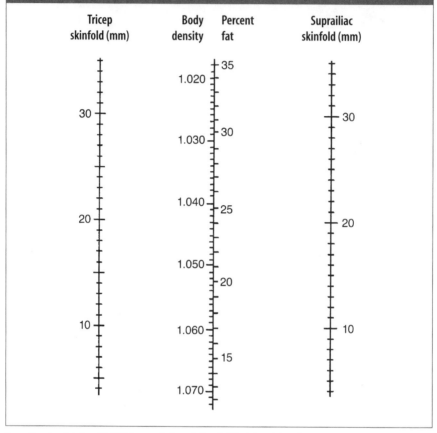

Source: Based on data from (1) A. W. Sloan et al., *Journal of Applied Physiology* 17 (1962): 967, and (2) J. F. Brozek et al., *Annals of the New York Academy of Science* 101 (1963): 113.

IMPROPER PROCEDURES: Not maintaining the fold with your left hand; placing the skinfold pinchers less than or more than a half inch from your fingers when taking the measure; taking longer than 2 seconds to read the caliper measurement.

Evaluating Flexibility

Flexibility assessment involves measuring the maximum range of motion at a joint. Flexibility can be affected by muscle, tendon, and ligament tightness,

Nomograms for Conversion of Skinfolds to Body Density[1]
and Percent Body Fat[2] (Men)

Subscapular skinfold (mm)	Body density	Percent fat	Thigh skinfold (mm)

```
Subscapular              Body    Percent              Thigh
skinfold (mm)           density    fat           skinfold (mm)

30                                                          30
                    1.030 ─┐─ 30
                    1.040 ─┤─ 25
20                  1.050 ─┤                                20
                           ┤─ 20
                    1.060 ─┤
                           ┤─ 15
                    1.070 ─┤
10                  1.080 ─┤─ 10                            10
                    1.090 ─┤─ 5
                    1.100 ─┘
```

which can limit movement about the joint. The loss of the ability to bend, twist, and stretch is often a result of muscle disuse, such as in excessive periods of sitting or standing. Sedentary living habits can lead to loss of flexibility, lower-back pain, and muscle imbalances. For example, shortening of the hamstrings (the muscles located in the back of the thighs) is very common. Extreme flexibility, however, has no advantage. If your joints are too loose or flexible, you may be more susceptible to joint injuries. Exercises for stretching the major muscle groups are discussed in Chapter 8. Although no single test will provide adequate information about the flexibility of all the major joints of

TABLE 3.1 Norms for Body Composition (% body fat)		
	Women	**Men**
Desirable	16 – 25	12 – 20
Overfat	25.1 – 34.9	20.1 – 24.9
Obese	⩾ 35	⩾ 25

your body, the following trunk flexion test is the most commonly used test and provides a reasonable indication of lower-back and hamstring flexibility. Refer to Table 3.2 for the norms for trunk flexion.

⁑ Trunk Flexion

PURPOSE: To measure the flexibility of your lower back and hamstrings.

EQUIPMENT: Ruler, 6- to 8-inch stairstep or bench, powder or chalk, masking tape.

SETUP: Place the ruler on the edge of the stairstep or bench so that the 6-inch mark is aligned with the edge. Tape the ruler in place.

PROCEDURE: Sit with your legs fully extended and the bottoms of your feet (shoes off) flat against the stairstep or bench, with the ruler between your feet (see Figure 3.4). Be careful not to knock the ruler loose. Put chalk or powder on your middle fingertips. Place your hands over the ruler, one hand on top of the other, aligning your middle fingers. Slowly exhale and extend (stretch) your arms and hands forward as far as possible while maintaining the finger alignment and straight legs. Allow your head to curl forward as you reach. Pause when you can reach no farther and tap the ruler with your chalked middle fingertip. Do not bounce to gain extra distance. Return to the starting position and deter-

TABLE 3.2 Norms for Trunk Flexion (inches)		
	Women	**Men**
Excellent	12+	12+
Good	11 – 12	9 – 12
Average	9 – 11	8 – 9
Fair	7 – 9	6 – 8
Poor	0 – 7	0 – 6

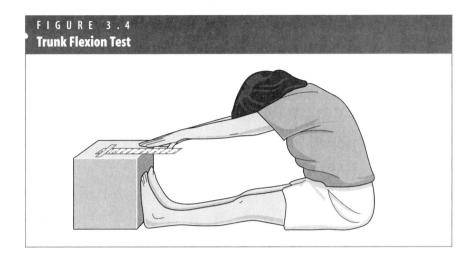

FIGURE 3.4
Trunk Flexion Test

mine where your fingertip touched the ruler. Read the ruler at the far-
thest edge of the chalk mark. Repeat two or three times and record your
best score.

IMPROPER PROCEDURES: Not maintaining middle-finger alignment; not paus-
ing in the full reach position (for example, bouncing to get extra distance); bending at the knees.

Evaluating Motor Skill

Although athletic skill and general motor skill are not health-related components of physical fitness, some of you may wish to test your abilities. Chapter
9 provides some advanced training strategies for those who wish to go beyond
the basic training for physical fitness and to improve their speed, agility, and
explosiveness. This section addresses three motor skill tests.

General motor skill refers to one's level of ability in a wide range of physical activities. Speed, power, balance, agility, reaction time, and coordination are
all components of motor skill performance. In a successful performance, these
skills blend into a single effective movement, such as stroking a tennis ball.
The movement may be quite complex. For example, hitting a forehand in tennis involves three moving factors: the ball, the body (feet), and the racquet.
Integration of motor skills in a coordinated manner leads to graceful and successful movement.

The skills involved in each sport are quite specific, and success in one activity does not necessarily mean equal success in another. In any case, it is impossible to measure all the specifics of complex physical activities. Thus an
acceptable alternative has been to sample some of the specific traits involved

TABLE 3.3
Norms for Motor Skills

	Agility Run (seconds)		20-Yard Dash (seconds)		Vertical Jump (inches)	
	Women	Men	Women	Men	Women	Men
Excellent	≤ 19.0	≤ 16.7	≤ 3.05	≤ 2.75	16+	24+
Good	19.1 – 20.4	16.8 – 17.3	3.10 – 3.20	2.80 – 2.90	14 – 15.5	22.5 – 23.5
Average	20.5 – 21.7	17.4 – 17.9	3.25 – 3.35	2.95 – 3.05	12.5 – 13.5	21.0 – 22.0
Fair	21.8 – 23.1	18.0 – 18.5	3.40 – 3.50	3.10 – 3.20	11.0 – 12.0	19.5 – 20.5
Poor	23.2+	18.6+	3.55+	3.25+	≤ 10.5	≤ 19.0

in athletic performance. A person who scores well on a motor skill test usually has the potential to succeed in a sport in which he or she receives instruction and practice.

The tests presented here do not examine all the traits related to general athletic ability. However, the agility run, 20-yard dash, and vertical jump are excellent indicators of agility, speed, and power, respectively. Again, based on the time needed to perform them and the ease of administering and scoring them, these tests are practical tools for getting a sense of your general athletic ability. Use Table 3.3 to rate your performance on the tests. You may find that you are not satisfied with your performance. In general, after some exercise training, it is easier to improve on the basic exercise tests than on tests of athletic skill. However, with some specific motor skill exercises, you can become faster, more agile, and more explosive. Use your test results as a starting point.

ᛁᚷ *Vertical Jump*

PURPOSE: To measure the muscular power of your lower extremities.

EQUIPMENT: Measuring tape, chalk or powder, step stool, masking tape.

SETUP: Find a room with a high ceiling and a section of wall with no obstructions. Tape the measuring tape to the wall using the masking tape (see Figure 3.5). The measuring tape should extend at least 10 feet from the floor (depending on how tall you are and how high you can jump). Place some chalk or powder on the fingertips of your middle fingers.

PROCEDURE: Face the wall with your feet flat on the floor and your toes touching the wall. Raise both arms overhead and fully extend, reaching as high as you can. Touch the wall with your fingertips, leaving a chalk mark. Now rechalk your fingertips and turn sideways to the wall. Without moving your feet (you are not allowed to step into the jump), swing

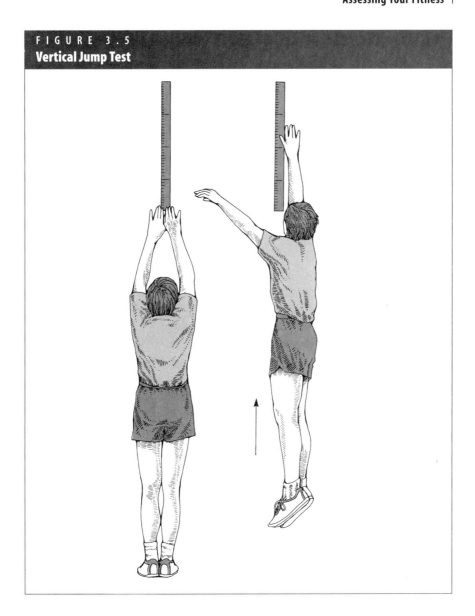

FIGURE 3.5
Vertical Jump Test

your arms down as you take a deep squat, then explosively swing your arms upward as you jump, touching the wall as high as possible with the fingers nearest the wall. After a brief rest, try a second jump. Record the greatest vertical distance (to the nearest half inch) obtained between your standing reach and your jumping reach. Refer to Table 3.3 for norms for the vertical jump.

IMPROPER PROCEDURES: Not measuring a true standing reach; moving your feet in preparing to jump.

20-Yard Dash

PURPOSE: To measure your movement speed and power.

EQUIPMENT: Stopwatch, masking tape, measuring tape.

SETUP: Measure off 20 yards (60 feet), and mark the beginning and end with masking tape.

PROCEDURE: For this test, it is best to have a partner to serve as timer. Have your partner stand at the finish line with one arm raised and the stopwatch in the raised hand. As he or she drops the raised hand, the stopwatch is started. Start running when you see the hand begin to drop, and sprint as fast as you can through the finish line. Record your times to the nearest tenth of a second for each of three trials. Refer to Table 3.3 for norms for the 20-yard dash.

IMPROPER PROCEDURES: Jumping the start signal; slowing down before you get to the finish line.

Agility Run

PURPOSE: To measure your quickness, speed, ability to change direction, and balance.

EQUIPMENT: Four chairs or boxes, timing device, masking tape, measuring tape.

SETUP: Refer to Figure 3.6. Use masking tape for the start and finish lines.

PROCEDURE: For this test, again, it is best to have a partner to serve as timer. Lie face down with your head just behind the starting line and your arms positioned as if you were about to perform a push-up. On the command "Go" (the stopwatch starts), jump to your feet and run as fast as you can to the end line, a distance of 30 feet. As one foot touches or crosses the end line, turn around and sprint back to the starting line. Next, weave in and out around the four chairs or boxes, without touching them, to the end line. Then turn and weave back through the chairs (in the opposite direction) to the starting line. Finally, sprint to the end line, touch or cross it with your foot, and and then turn and sprint back to the starting line. Record your time to the nearest tenth of a second. Refer to Table 3.3 for norms for the agility run.

IMPROPER PROCEDURES: Not touching or crossing the lines at each end; touching a chair or box; not following the prescribed course.

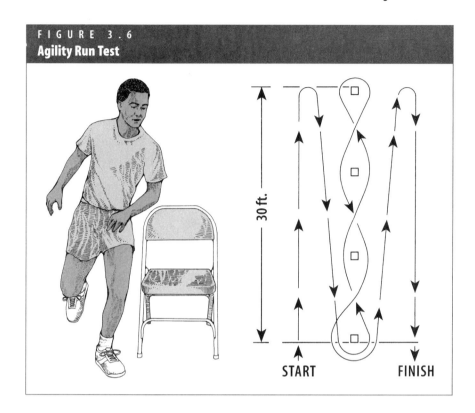

FIGURE 3.6
Agility Run Test

30 ft.

START   FINISH

Evaluating Muscular Strength

Strength is traditionally measured by determining your 1 repetition maximum (1 RM), which is the amount of weight you can lift only one time. We recommend that beginners use resistance machines (Universal, Nautilus, Cybex) rather than free weights (barbells, dumbbells) to test strength. *If you are using free weights, someone must be present to help with the testing.* The two tests discussed here measure muscular strength of the upper and lower body. Specifically the chest press test measures the muscular strength of the chest, shoulders, and arms, while the leg press measures the muscular strength of the hips and thighs. People often take strength for granted, as if it were something we are born with. However, building and maintaining muscular strength throughout life takes commitment and work.

Because strength can be greatly affected by one's size, the strength data in Table 3.4 are relative strength measures. In other words, to compare your numbers with those in the table, you have to divide your 1 RM by your body weight. For example, Sue's bench press is 100 pounds, and she weighs 120 pounds.

WAY OF LIFE
Predicting Your 1 RM

- An alternative to directly determining your 1 RM is to predict it using a weight that you can lift 2 to 10 times. Use the following formula to predict 1 RM:

$$\text{predicted 1 RM (lbs.)} = \frac{\text{weight lifted}}{0.935 - ([\text{no. of reps.} - 2] \times 0.025)}$$

Thus Sue's relative strength is 100 divided by 120, or 0.83. According to Table 3.4, her chest press strength is excellent.

⚇ *Chest Press*

PURPOSE: To determine the strength of the muscles of your chest, shoulders, and arms.

EQUIPMENT: Chest press machine or, alternatively, a bench, bar, and weights.

SETUP: Prior to beginning the testing, perform a 3- to 5-minute warm-up involving movements of the legs and arms. After the warm-up, lie back on the bench and position your hands about shoulder width apart on the handles. Slide up or down on the bench so that your hands are positioned about nipple level and your elbows are directly under the handles. Your feet should be firmly planted on the floor at slightly wider than shoulder width, and your back should be flat on the bench.

TABLE 3.4
Norms for Muscular Strength Relative to Body Weight (1 RM/body weight)

| | Women | | Men | |
	Chest Press	Leg Press	Chest Press	Leg Press
Excellent	⩾ 0.81	⩾ 1.75	⩾ 1.31	⩾ 2.30
Good	0.75 – 0.80	1.45 – 1.74	1.11 – 1.30	2.10 – 2.29
Average	0.70 – 0.74	1.31 – 1.44	1.00 – 1.10	2.00 – 2.09
Fair	0.41 – 0.69	1.00 – 1.30	0.50 – 0.99	1.61 – 1.99
Poor	⩽ 0.40	⩽ 0.99	⩽ 0.49	⩽ 1.60

PROCEDURE: Place a very light weight on the machine, and perform 5 to 10 practice lifts. After the practice lifts, place a weight that you feel you can lift once on the machine. As a rule of thumb, a good starting weight is 70 percent and 100 percent of body weight for women and men, respectively. Position yourself on the bench (see the test setup), and attempt the lift. If the attempt was successful, add more weight; if it was unsuccessful, remove some weight. Take a 3-minute rest and perform another attempt. Continue this process until you have determined your 1 RM. (*Note:* The goal is to determine the 1 RM in as few attempts as possible, so use your best judgment when increasing or decreasing the weight after attempts.) Refer to Table 3.4 for norms for the chest press.

IMPROPER PROCEDURES: Holding your breath; not maintaining proper form while performing the lift; arching your lower back; lifting your buttocks off the bench; lifting one or both feet off the floor; twisting your torso on the bench.

⅄ *Leg Press*

PURPOSE: To determine the strength of the muscles of your hips and thighs.

EQUIPMENT: Leg press machine.

SETUP: We assume that you have already warmed up prior to performing the chest press. If not, then do so now (see the chest press setup). Adjust the machine so that at its lowest position, your knees make a 90-degree angle.

PROCEDURE: Place a very light weight on the machine and perform 5 to 10 practice lifts. After the practice lifts, place a weight that you feel you can lift once on the machine. As a rule of thumb, a good starting weight is 130 percent and 200 percent of body weight for women and men, respectively. Position yourself on the leg press machine (see the test setup), and attempt the lift. If the attempt was successful, add more weight; if unsuccessful, remove some weight. Take a 3-minute rest, and perform another attempt. Continue this process until you have determined your 1 RM. (*Note:* The goal is to determine the 1 RM in as few attempts as possible, so use your best judgment when increasing or decreasing the weight after attempts.) Refer to Table 3.4 for norms for the leg press.

IMPROPER PROCEDURES: Holding your breath; not maintaining proper form while performing the lift; lifting your buttocks off the seat or pad; not going deep enough (less than a 90-degree knee angle) during the press.

Evaluating Muscular Endurance

The two tests discussed here measure the muscular endurance of key major muscle groups of the body. The push-up test assesses the muscular endurance of the muscles of the chest, arms, and shoulders. The abdominal crunch test measures the muscular endurance of the abdominal muscles. The abdominal muscles play an important role in maintaining correct posture, thus reducing the risk for lower-back pain. Additionally the abdominal muscles have been described as the center of strength. Working in conjunction with the back extensor muscles, the abdominal muscles stabilize the torso to provide a rigid base around which the muscles of the extremities can apply force. These muscles play a vital role in many daily activities.

Remember, the purpose of these tests is to help you assess your muscular endurance and, most important, to determine your own baseline for future comparison.

⁖⅄ Push-ups

PURPOSE: To test the muscular endurance of the muscles of your chest, arms, and shoulders.

EQUIPMENT: Timing device.

PROCEDURE: Kneel on all fours, with your hands about shoulder width apart and positioned beneath your shoulders. Extend your legs back, with the weight on your toes and your body in a straight line. As you bend at the elbows, lower your body as a unit until you achieve a 90-degree bend at the elbows. Keeping your back straight, press yourself to the up position. Repeat this procedure for 1 minute.

(*Note:* If you are unable to perform one standard pushup, your muscular endurance is poor. In order to establish a baseline measure with this test, use a modified push-up. Kneel on all fours, with your hands about shoulder width apart and positioned beneath your shoulders. Extend your legs back, but this time, place your weight on your bent knees, with your body in a straight line. As you bend at the elbows, lower your body as a unit until you achieve a 90-degree bend at the elbows. Keeping your back straight, press yourself to the up position.) Refer to Table 3.5 for norms for push-ups.

IMPROPER PROCEDURES: Not keeping your body straight, allowing it to sag or peak upwards; not going down to a 90-degree elbow bend; failing to fully straighten your arms when pressing back up.

TABLE 3.5 Norms for Muscular Endurance				
	Women*		Men*	
	Crunches	Push-ups	Crunches	Push-ups
Excellent	45+	24+	54+	40+
Good	39 – 44	16 – 23	46 – 43	34 – 39
Average	31 – 38	10 – 15	41 – 45	28 – 33
Fair	26 – 30	4 – 9	36 – 40	22 – 27
Poor	0 – 25	0 – 3	0 – 35	0 – 21

*Norms for standard push-up.

Abdominal Crunches

PURPOSE: To determine the muscular endurance of the abdominal muscles.

EQUIPMENT: Exercise mat, two cardboard pieces (3 by 6 inches), masking tape, ruler, timing device.

SETUP: Align the cardboard pieces with the mat's edge about hip width apart (see Figure 3.7), and secure them to the mat with masking tape.

PROCEDURE: Lie on your back with your arms straight and resting on the floor by your side. The palms of your hands should be turned down toward the floor. Position your body so that your fingertips just touch the leading edge of the cardboard pieces. Draw your feet back toward your buttocks until they are flat on the floor (knees bent). The angle of your legs to your thighs should be approximately 90 degrees. Just prior to beginning the test, round your lower back so that it touches the mat, maintaining contact throughout the test. Tuck your chin to your chest. Contract your abdominal muscles, lifting your shoulder blades while sliding your hands along the cardboard pieces until your fingertips touch the edge of the mat. Your hands must remain in contact with the cardboard throughout the crunching movement. Return to the starting position and repeat this procedure as many times as possible within 1 minute. Resting is permitted, but only in the starting position. Refer to Table 3.5 for norms for abdominal crunches.

IMPROPER PROCEDURES: Not crunching enough to reach the end of the mat; not returning to the starting position between repetitions; holding your breath during the test.

> ### FIGURE 3.7
> **Abdominal Crunches**

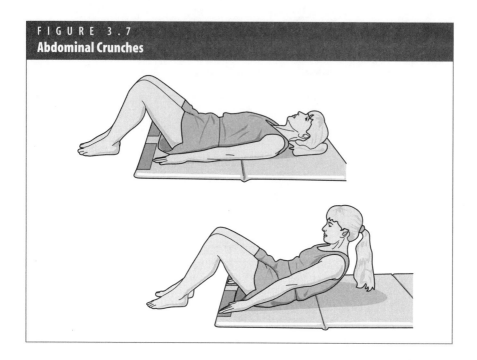

Evaluating Cardiorespiratory Endurance

As discussed in Chapter 1, cardiorespiratory endurance depends on the ability of the heart to pump blood, the lungs to breathe volumes of air, and the muscles to utilize oxygen. Therefore sustained muscular activity is possible only through their effective functioning. Various tests involving vigorous physical movement that make increased demands on the heart and lungs have been devised to assess cardiorespiratory endurance.

Procedures for determining aerobic capacity (cardiorespiratory endurance) in the laboratory are complex, time-consuming, and impractical for testing large numbers of people. Recent studies, therefore, have attempted to develop **field tests** that can be substituted for laboratory tests. Field tests like the 1.5-mile run and the step test have correlated well with laboratory-determined values for cardiorespiratory endurance. Thus field tests make it quite easy to determine your cardiorespiratory endurance and to detect changes due to training. The 1.5-mile run and the step test described are commonly used to assess cardiorespiratory endurance. If you are in fairly good shape and are comfortable jogging or running, then perform the 1.5-mile run. However, if you are sedentary and not comfortable running, then perform the step test. Both will give you a good indication of your cardiorespiratory endurance.

☺ 1.5-Mile Run

Most field tests of cardiorespiratory endurance utilize running or walking. Bruno Balke, a physician-physiologist, has demonstrated that an adequate estimate of aerobic capacity (cardiorespiratory endurance) is possible after as little as 10 minutes of running at a near maximal effort. If the runs are completed in less than 8 to 10 minutes, a significant amount of energy comes from anaerobic sources. But if maximum work is performed for 10 to 20 minutes, the energy comes predominantly from the utilization of oxygen. Therefore distance runs of 1.5 miles, which typically take 10 to 20 minutes to complete, are valid cardiorespiratory endurance field tests, especially for those who have some experience in running.

PURPOSE: To test the capability of your respiratory and cardiovascular systems to meet the energy demands of your body during aerobic activity.

EQUIPMENT: Timing device.

SETUP: Measure a 1.5-mile course, or locate a high school/university track.

PROCEDURES: After a 3- to 5-minute warm-up (see Chapter 4), measure the time it takes to run the 1.5 miles. Pacing is very important. You do not want to start out running and finish walking, nor do you want to start too slow and finish with energy left over. Try to maintain a consistent running pace that allows you to complete the course in a minimum amount of time. Refer to Table 3.6 for norms for the 1.5-mile run. If you are not accustomed to running or do not feel you can run the entire 1.5 miles, then use the step test to assess your cardiorespiratory endurance.

IMPROPER PROCEDURES: Not finishing the 1.5-mile course.

TABLE 3.6
Norms for Cardiorespiratory Endurance

	Women		Men	
	1.5 Mile Run (minutes)	**Step Test (bpm)**	**1.5 Mile Run (minutes)**	**Step Test (bpm)**
Excellent	≤ 13:00	≤ 135	≤ 10:45	≤ 132
Good	13:01 – 14:19	136 – 153	10:46 – 11:30	133 – 147
Average	14:20 – 15:38	154 – 170	11:31 – 12:15	148 – 162
Fair	15:39 – 16:57	171 – 187	12:16 – 13:00	163 – 177
Poor	16:58+	188+	13:01+	178+

⚝ Step Test

Another useful procedure for assessing your cardiorespiratory endurance is the step test, a heart-rate recovery measure. Stepping on and off a bench for a 3- to 5-minute time period at a selected cadence has long been used for rating a person's physical capacity for hard work and for evaluating the effects of training. Although not considered the best measure of cardiorespiratory endurance, the heart rate during recovery from a standardized step test is a simple way to evaluate the heart's response to exercise. The faster your heart rate recovers after the standardized exercise bout, the higher your fitness rating. The test is easy to administer on an individual basis or to a large group. It takes little time, does not require special skills to perform, and requires a minimum of equipment.

PURPOSE: To indirectly assess your cardiorespiratory endurance based on your heart rate recovery.

EQUIPMENT: 16- to 18-inch bench (or sturdy chair, locker room bench, bleachers), timing device, and metronome. (*Note:* If metronome is not available, practice repeating "up up down down" in 2-second intervals.)

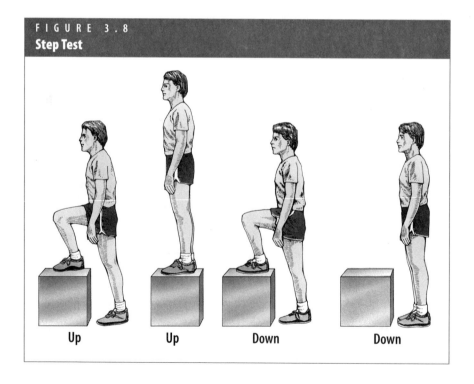

FIGURE 3.8
Step Test

| Up | Up | Down | Down |

PROCEDURE: Start the metronome, which should be set at 120 beats per minute. Start the timing device with your first step beginning with the left foot up, then the right foot up, then the left foot down, and then the right foot down (see Figure 3.8). This four-count sequence represents one complete step. At 120 beats per minute, you will execute 30 steps per minute. It is permissible to change the "up" foot during the test. Continue the test for 3 minutes, keeping tempo with the metronome. Be sure to straighten your knees as you step up onto the bench.

Upon completion of the 3 minutes of stepping, begin your recovery period by sitting on a chair or straddling the bench and resting quietly. One minute into the recovery period, count your pulse for 30 seconds (for example, 1:00 to 1:30), and record it. Repeat this procedure for the second (2:00 to 2:30) and third (3:00 to 3:30) minutes of recovery. To take your pulse, press lightly with your index and middle fingers on the inside of your wrist on the thumb side or just below the jawbone in the hollow beside the Adam's apple (see Chapter 5 for more detailed instructions on how to take your pulse).

To determine your recovery index, sum the three 30-second pulse measurements and compare your personal recovery index for the step test with the norms in Table 3.6.

IMPROPER PROCEDURES: Not keeping the cadence of 30 step executions per minute; failing to straighten your knees to full extension on the up steps; not counting your pulse accurately.

Using Your Results to Develop Your Own Fitness Profile

Once you have evaluated your fitness or skill level for each component, use the information as a starting point for developing your personal fitness program. It is not unusual to find that you possess strengths in some areas and weaknesses in others. Very few individuals have excellent levels of fitness for every fitness component, yet all of us should strive to reach our full potential in them all. For example, if you rate "excellent" for cardiorespiratory endurance, either maintain your current fitness program or try cross-training or advanced training for a little "spice" (see Chapter 9). But if your muscular strength and endurance assessments showed a poor fitness profile, build your program around the suggestions for beginners in Chapter 7.

After you have participated regularly in any program for approximately six weeks, you may wish to perform these self-assessments once again to measure any improvements made. Of course, you should feel and see improvements after undertaking a fitness program. However, actually measuring these changes adds motivation. On the other hand, if you do not see even slight improvements in the areas your fitness program has concentrated on, it is time to reevaluate your approach. Make certain you are following all guidelines suggested in this book. Refer to the specific chapters on each fitness component and make workout adjustments. Continue to regularly reassess until you reach your goals. Periodically (for example, yearly) perform the assessments to make certain you are not slipping, to motivate and reward your hard work, and to remind yourself how far you have come.

Summary

Measurement and evaluation are very important in our everyday lives. How many miles to the gallon of gasoline do we get? Which product is the better buy? How does a professor rate as a teacher? We continuously measure and evaluate various facets of our daily living. Through the use of objective physical fitness tests, you can evaluate your own physical fitness. The tests discussed in this chapter are all easily administered and provide useful ratings of the physical fitness of men and women. The success of the testing program, however, depends on careful and accurate administration of the tests.

Testing should not dominate your exercise program, but it can be a worthwhile motivator to greater effort and to regular, desirable exercise habits. It is also natural to be curious about how you compare with others. The tables in this chapter allow you to see where you stand based on your test results and will give you greater insight into your physical strengths and weaknesses. Use this information to develop your individualized physical fitness program. The following chapters examine the benefits and training specifics for improving and maintaining optimal cardiorespiratory endurance, muscular strength and endurance, flexibility, and body composition.

Key Words

FAT WEIGHT: The absolute amount of body fat, usually expressed in pounds.

FIELD TESTS: Tests that take place outside the laboratory.

LEAN BODY WEIGHT: The absolute amount of lean body tissue, usually expressed in pounds. Muscle, bone, and organ tissue make up the majority of lean body tissue.

SKINFOLD CALIPERS: An instrument used in body composition assessment to measure the thickness of a fold of skin and its underlying, or subcutaneous, fat.

TEST BATTERY: A series of tests used to measure the various components of physical fitness.

A Way of Life Library

MacDougall, H. A., N. K. Wenger, and H. J. Green. *Physiological Testing of the High-Performance Athlete.* Champaign, IL: Human Kinetics,1991.

Maud, P. J., and C. Foster. *Physiological Assessment of Human Fitness.* Champaign, IL: Human Kinetics, 1995.

Morrow, J. R., A. W. Jackson, J. F. Disch, and D. P. Mood. *Measurement and Evaluation in Human Performance.* Champaign, IL: Human Kinetics, 1995.

Winnick, J. P., and F. X. Short. *Physical Fitness Testing of the Disabled.* Champaign, IL: Human Kinetics, 1985.

CHAPTER 4

The Basic Principles of Exercise

This chapter provides the framework for assisting you in developing a personalized exercise program. In recent years, advances in exercise and sports science have led to the development of sound

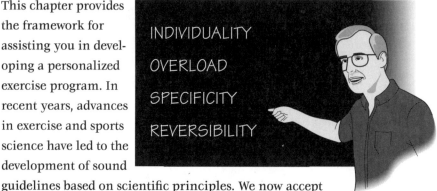

INDIVIDUALITY

OVERLOAD

SPECIFICITY

REVERSIBILITY

guidelines based on scientific principles. We now accept that exercise must be prescribed on an individual basis. Also, we now recognize that any physical fitness program must involve a balance of training for cardiorespiratory endurance, muscular strength and endurance, flexibility, and body composition. In this chapter, we are primarily concerned with the basic principles used to design your personal exercise program. The specifics for developing a training program for each component of physical fitness will be discussed in later chapters. Note that these principles are applicable regardless of your age or present physical condition. The key is learning to regulate your workouts based on your body's response to the exercise work load.

As you read this chapter, keep these statements in mind:

- Your body will become stronger as you exercise at a greater-than-normal level.
- It takes effort to be physically fit; however, your training program does not have to be punishing to reap physiological benefits.
- Adaptations to training are specific and limited to the muscles and physiological systems involved in the exercise.
- Muscular strength and endurance activities, flexibility activities, and cardiorespiratory training should be combined in a regular program.

- A workout for developing physical fitness consists of three essential parts: a warm-up, a vigorous conditioning period, and a cool-down.
- After each workout, you should feel refreshed and relaxed, rather than uncomfortable and exhausted. Prolonged fatigue lasting for more than an hour following your workout probably means your workout was too demanding.
- Exercise can lead to injuries. Quite often an injury is the result of overdoing it. When beginning a program, start out slowly and progress gradually in order to prevent unnecessary injuries.

It is imperative to understand how to begin and how to progress from a light to a more strenuous workout. Without a clear understanding of the exercise principles, you might embark on a sporadic, unsafe, and ineffective training program, resulting in unnecessary soreness, frustration, discouragement, and possibly injury. This chapter will help you establish a personal system for regulating your workouts. The basic exercise principles presented here apply equally well to men and women regardless of age or physical condition. And proper application of these principles will allow you to structure a fitness program to suit your precise physical needs.

PRINCIPLE 1

The Individuality Principle
The training program should be designed around you.

No one program can be designed to accommodate everyone because we all differ in terms of initial fitness levels, physical attributes, physical limitations, and training goals. Just because we are all interested in having healthy cardiorespiratory systems does not mean that everyone can simply go out and perform the same training program. Even the popular exercise videotapes that seem to be designed for everyone warn that you should exercise at your own pace and perform only those movements within your capabilities. Another analogy would be to say that anyone interested in getting stronger should start a training program by performing the bench press with 100 pounds. This would be too light for some, just right for a few, and crushing to others.

The purpose of undergoing the various fitness assessments outlined in Chapter 3 was to help you ascertain your current fitness levels and increase your awareness of which fitness components need improvement. Before embarking on a training program, you should reexamine your results in the various assessments. In addition, you should write down your reasons for starting or continuing an exercise program. Then prioritize your reasons. Armed

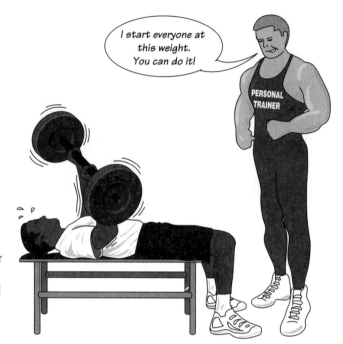

There is no one set program that works for everyone. The best programs are designed around your strengths and weaknesses.

with your testing results and your priority list, you can individualize your training by designing a program that meets your specific fitness goals. Following the individuality principle not only will help you start a successful exercise program but also will help you maintain the program. People's lives are always in a state of flux, and so their exercise programs should be as well. Injuries, illnesses, or changes in fitness goals—all will require you to routinely reassess your program. Designing and/or upgrading a program in this fashion will help enhance its efficacy and provide great positive reinforcement as you work toward your goals.

PRINCIPLE 2
The Overload Principle
The training program should be taxing to your body.

To improve your physical fitness, you must ask your body to do something it is not used to doing on a regular basis. The body is not challenged by activities to which it is accustomed. Thus a properly designed training program must incorporate regular training at intensities that challenge the body. Fortunately the overload doesn't have to be punishing or exhaustive. Intensity, duration, and

WAY OF LIFE
Training Variables Associated with the Overload Principle

- *Intensity*—How hard?
- *Duration*—How long?
- *Frequency*—How often?

frequency are the three training variables associated with the overload principle that can be adjusted to control the level of difficulty of your fitness program.

Intensity: Difficulty of the Workout

Intensity refers to how hard the training is. The higher the intensity, the more strenuous the training. The intensity of a training program is gauged differently depending on the nature of the exercise. For example, the intensity of a cardiorespiratory training program is generally based on **exercise heart rate** (see the Karvonen method in Chapter 5). The higher the heart rate, the more intense the workout. For strength training, the intensity is based on the amount

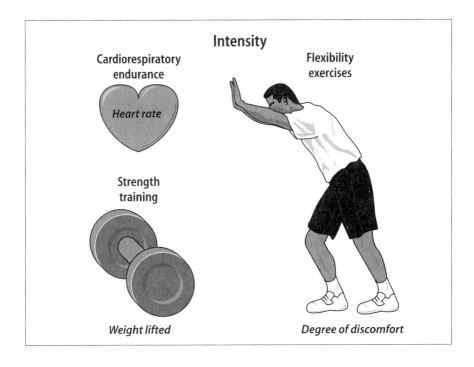

Intensity

Cardiorespiratory
endurance

Heart rate

Flexibility
exercises

Strength
training

Weight lifted

Degree of discomfort

of weight lifted. The intensity for each flexibility exercise is based on the degree of discomfort experienced while stretching. Specifics on intensity for each type of training will be discussed in the following chapters.

Duration: Length of the Workout

Duration refers to the length of time the body is actually being overloaded during a training workout. The duration of a workout varies depending on the type of exercise being performed. Cardiorespiratory exercise should have a duration of 20 to 60 minutes of continuous activity. Duration of strength training is measured by the number of sets and repetitions performed. For flexibility, the duration is determined by the amount of time the stretch is held and the total number of stretches performed. Specifics on the duration required for each type of training will be discussed in subsequent chapters.

Frequency: Number of Workouts

Frequency refers to the number of times (usually on a per week basis) that you work out. As with intensity and duration, the frequency of training varies with the type of training and the goals of your fitness program. Cardiorespiratory training is usually performed three to five times per week, while strength training is performed two to three times per week. Flexibility training can be

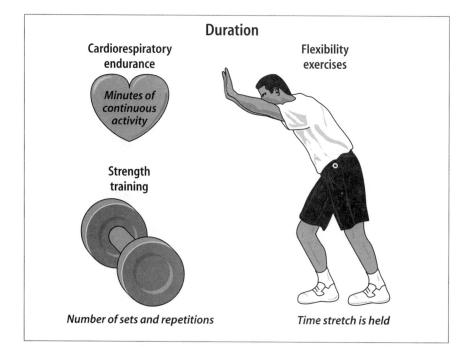

Duration

Cardiorespiratory endurance

Minutes of continuous activity

Strength training

Flexibility exercises

Number of sets and repetitions

Time stretch is held

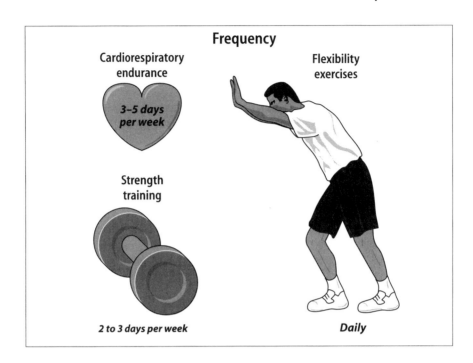

performed seven times per week. Again, specifics on the frequency for each type of exercise will be discussed in the following chapters.

As already stated, adjusting one, two, or all three of these variables will affect the training overload. Learning to manipulate these training variables will enable you to make fitness improvements or to maintain your fitness throughout life.

PRINCIPLE 3
The Specificity Principle
Training adaptations are highly specific.

The human body adapts in a very specific manner to the demands placed upon it by training. These adaptations are biomechanically, anatomically, and physiologically specific—specific to body positioning, the joint angles and range of motion used during training, the muscles involved, and the nature (for instance, speed and duration) of the movements performed during training. For example, running does little to improve your performance in biking even though you are using many of the same muscles. Why? Because biomechanically, the muscles are being used differently in the two activities. Also, although running will cause large increases in the muscular endurance of the leg muscles, the anatomical specificity of run training leads to little improvement in upper-body

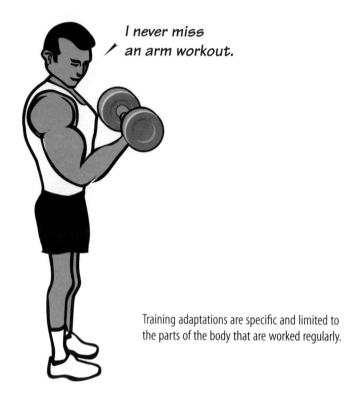

I never miss an arm workout.

Training adaptations are specific and limited to the parts of the body that are worked regularly.

muscular endurance. Physiological specificity tells us that running for improved cardiorespiratory endurance does little to cause changes in leg muscle strength. Why? Because the physiological demands placed on the leg muscles during endurance training are different from those of strength training. Likewise endurance run training does not increase sprinting ability. Again, physiological specificity indicates that the speed with which a muscle contracts and the energy it requires are different for endurance training and sprint training.

The specificity principle is one reason elite athletes must concentrate on one sport or activity. Their program must be designed to elicit the sport-specific adaptations that will enhance all aspects of performance. This explains why no one athlete can dominate in all sports. Although there are great heptathletes and decathletes, none reach the levels of sport performance that the single-event specialists do. Obviously no one training program could adequately prepare an athlete for the variety of demands required by the different sports.

However, training for general fitness is much different than training for the specialized demands of sport participation. A general fitness training program should be designed to improve all the components of physical fitness. As a result, keep in mind the importance of participating in a balanced fitness program with an emphasis on fitness components that demonstrate a weakness.

For example, if your fitness goal is to improve your muscular strength, then prioritize your training accordingly. This does not mean that you stop training for cardiorespiratory endurance, but rather that you spend more of your training time working on muscular strength and less on cardiorespiratory endurance. Simply changing the order in which you train can be enough. In other words, training for strength before you go out for a run would be a way of prioritizing your training for the greatest improvements in strength. A word of warning: You should not prioritize your training to the extent that you stop training for the other fitness components (see the reversibility principle). Training programs designed with the specificity principle in mind allow you to achieve your ever-changing fitness goals.

PRINCIPLE 4
The Reversibility Principle
Fitness is for life and so should be your training.

Regular exercise enables you to improve and maintain your fitness capabilities. But if your workouts are sporadic or stop altogether, your fitness level will drop to a level that only meets the demands of daily living. Simply stated, the reversibility principle says that if you don't use it, you lose it. In other words, if

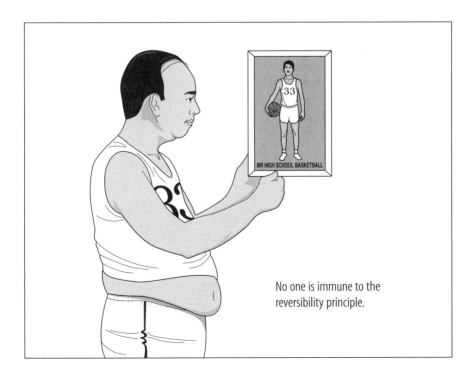

No one is immune to the reversibility principle.

you stop training, you will begin to lose the training adaptations you worked so hard for. This is why we say fitness is for life. Training is not something you do three months out of the year in order to get ready for swimsuit weather. It is something you do year round. Although your reasons for training will certainly change as you go through life, it is critical that you adapt your training program without interrupting its regularity. Knowledge of the training principles will help you to do so and enable you to enjoy the benefits of an effective lifelong fitness program.

Elements of a Workout

Very few people have the ability, the time and lifestyle, or the desire to achieve the level of physical fitness of an Olympic competitor. Still, anyone who wishes to maximize their fitness potential on a more realistic level can certainly do so. The goal of this book is to help you reach and maintain a level of physical fitness that is in step with your everyday living habits. The following elements of a workout apply to training programs geared for everyone from Olympic-caliber athletes to those of us who simply want to make physical fitness a way of life.

The Three-Segment Workout

Many workouts for developing and maintaining physical fitness consist of three essential parts: a warm-up, a conditioning period, and a cool-down. All three segments are particularly essential for a sound cardiorespiratory endurance program.

The Warm-up

A proper **warm-up** before each workout is a wise habit. It prepares you mentally and physically for the vigorous training segment of the workout. Warming up can serve as a precaution against unnecessary injuries and muscle soreness. It stimulates the heart and lungs moderately and progressively, and it increases the blood flow to the working muscles. The increased flow of warm blood into the muscles increases muscle temperature—thus the label "warm-up." As a general rule, walking and in some cases slow jogging are good choices to help you warm up. After 3 to 5 minutes of such exercise, it is common practice to do some range-of-motion movements at the major joints. Stretching the muscles and tendons prior to vigorous training can help prepare your body for the more forceful contractions performed during the conditioning segment. However, *do not confuse stretching with warming up. The act of stretching in and of itself does little to increase muscle temperature.*

The time required for warm-up varies with the individual. However, as soon as you begin to sweat (an indication that the temperature of the deep tis-

WAY OF LIFE
Elements of a Workout

- *Warm-up:* light general movements, stretching
- *Conditioning period:* cardiorespiratory and/or resistance exercises
- *Cool-down:* light general movements, stretching

sues has increased), you are probably ready for the more intense conditioning segment of the workout. You should keep in mind that cool weather requires longer warm-up times.

The Conditioning Period

After sufficient warm-up, you are ready for the main **conditioning period** of your workout. This is the period of time in which the body is vigorously worked. The conditioning period can consist of any physically challenging activity as long as the frequency, intensity, and duration are sufficient to cause a training response. Activities such as walking, running, bicycling, swimming, aerobics, calisthenics, resistance training, interval training, and circuit training are all possible training activities. Combinations of various activities can also be used during the conditioning segment; this cross-training adds variety and enjoyment to your workout. On some days, vigorous participation in your favorite sport may be used as the conditioning activity. The key is to make sure your intensity of training is sufficient to stimulate your body to adapt. In the following chapters, we examine the training intensities required for the various modes of exercise.

The Cool-down

The **cool-down** is the tapering-off of activity upon completion of the vigorous conditioning period. The activities performed during the cool-down vary depending on the type of activity used in the conditioning period. For example, after strength training, the cool-down may consist of slow and controlled movements mimicking those used in training combined with stretching. But a cool-down segment is not normally needed after flexibility training.

For cardiorespiratory training, the cool-down may be a continuation of activity at a progressively lower intensity. The cool-down prevents the pooling of blood in the extremities and enables the cardiorespiratory system to slowly return to resting levels. The light muscle activity of the cool-down assists in returning blood from the extremities to the heart. If you end a workout abruptly, your heart will continue to send extra blood to the muscles for a few minutes. Because the muscles are no longer contracting and helping to propel blood back to the heart, the blood pools in the extremities. In some cases, the blood pooling can cause dizziness and fainting after a workout. Generally a 5- to 10-minute cool-down period is sufficient. For most participants, the heart rate at the end of the cool-down should be below 100.

We recommend that you stretch toward the end of the cool-down segment, when your muscles are warm and pliable. The increased muscle elasticity allows for a greater range of motion about the joints and thus greater potential for improvements in flexibility.

Summary

Most people recognize the virtues of physical fitness, yet many of these same people do not maintain a regular fitness program. Two reasons for this failure to maintain individual fitness are not knowing how to design an exercise program and not knowing how to structure an actual workout session. You can be as creative in your program design as you want to be as long as you take into consideration the overload, specificity, individuality, and reversibility training principles. In doing so, you guarantee your program's effectiveness.

Each workout has three components. The conditioning segment is the foundation of any exercise program and can involve any activity or group of activities that stimulate and develop the various components of fitness. It's also important to engage in light muscular and stretching exercises during the warm-up and cool-down. Knowledge of the training principles and a properly structured workout will help make your fitness program adaptable, enjoyable, and, most important, rewarding.

Key Words

CONDITIONING PERIOD: The portion of a workout in which the body is vigorously exercised. The conditioning period can consist of any physically challenging activity as long as the frequency, intensity, and duration are sufficient to cause a training response.

COOL-DOWN: The last element of a workout consisting of a tapering-off in exercise intensity. The cool-down should include light general-type activity along with stretching exercises.

DURATION: A training variable associated with the overload principle that denotes the length of the workout session. The duration of a workout varies depending on the type of training being performed.

EXERCISE HEART RATE: A heart-beat rate (or pulse rate) per minute during exercise.

FREQUENCY: A training variable associated with the overload principle that refers to the number of times (usually on a per week basis) training is performed.

INTENSITY: A training variable associated with the overload principle that refers to how hard the training is. The intensity of a training program is gauged differently depending on the nature of the exercise. For example, cardiorespiratory exercise intensity is determined based on heart rate.

WARM-UP: The beginning element of a workout that prepares your body for more vigorous exercise. Generally walking and stretching of the major muscle groups are done during the warm-up period.

A *Way of Life Library*

American College of Sports Medicine. *ACSM Fitness Book*. Champaign, IL: Human Kinetics, 1992.
Fleck, S. J., and W. J. Kraemer. *Designing Resistance Training Programs*. Champaign, IL: Human Kinetics, 1987.
Franks, B. D., and E. T. Howley. *Fitness Facts*. Champaign, IL: Human Kinetics, 1989.

CHAPTER **5**

Developing Cardiorespiratory Endurance

Suppose you had to name the most important muscle in your body. Which one would
you choose? If you said the heart, you
already recognize the necessity for
optimal cardiorespiratory endurance.
This chapter focuses on how to plan a
program for developing and maintaining cardiorespiratory endurance. Such a
program conditions the heart, lungs, and
blood vessels and improves their ability to deliver oxygen to the muscle
tissue. *Continuous, rhythmic activities
that can be sustained over a period of 20
minutes or more are the best activities for
improving the functioning of the cardiorespiratory system.* Walking and running are convenient exercise modes with which to begin.
Bicycling, swimming, and other continuous
exertions also can provide an adequate stimulus for developing cardiorespiratory endurance and will be discussed in detail in Chapter 6. If
you are beginning an exercise program, it is important to start out at a
low level. As you advance, you will find it easy to adjust to higher levels of
exercise without undue fatigue.

As you read this chapter, keep these statements in mind:
- The types of exercise best suited to improving and maintaining cardiorespiratory endurance are also those best suited for achieving and maintaining
ideal levels of body fat.
- In order to improve cardiorespiratory endurance and body composition, a
vigorous overload is necessary.

- The exercise heart rate provides a reasonable indication of the intensity of a cardiorespiratory workout.
- Exercise programs involving continuous and rhythmic movements at an intensity of 50 to 85 percent of heart-rate reserve, for 20 to 60 minutes, three to five days per week, will provide significant improvements in cardiorespiratory endurance and thus the functioning of the heart, lungs, and blood vessels.

Benefits of Cardiorespiratory Exercise

The benefits of cardiorespiratory exercise are many. Healthy functioning of the cardiorespiratory system is of paramount importance for the maintenance of physical fitness and health. The continuous and rhythmic forms of exercise discussed in this chapter help reduce the risk for cardiorespiratory disease and premature death. Furthermore, activities that vigorously stimulate the heart and lungs over a period of time and that require plenty of oxygen strengthen the pumping ability of the heart, improve breathing capacity, and enhance the use of energy in the skeletal muscles. Each cell in our bodies needs a ready supply of oxygen and food, while carbon dioxide and other waste products must be carried away. Exercise improves the circulatory system's (the heart and blood vessels) ability to circulate blood throughout the body. The respiratory system (the lungs and air passages) becomes better at removing carbon dioxide and replacing it with fresh oxygen. The exercised heart, lungs, and muscles gradually function at a higher level both during physical exertion and at rest. These improvements are referred to as the **training effect.**

The training effect of cardiorespiratory exercise manifests itself in many ways. For example, the cardiac output (amount of blood pumped per minute by the heart) at rest is approximately the same for those who exercise regularly as for those who do not. Although there is no change in cardiac output after a period of endurance-type training (six to eight weeks), there is generally a reduction in the resting heart rate. The heart pumps more blood with each beat and does not have to beat as often to supply the body with blood. *It has become a more effective pump.* In addition, the slower heart rate allows the heart to rest longer between beats. The magnitude of this decrease in resting heart rate is dependent not only on the length of time you have been training but also on the intensity and amount of training. Imagine that after a couple of months of exercise training, you were able to lower your average per-minute heart rate by 10 beats. This would mean that your heart was beating 14,400 fewer times a day. A relatively slow heart rate, coupled with the greater volume of blood pumped per beat, makes for an efficient circulatory system.

During vigorous activity, the exercising muscles need increased amounts of oxygen to produce energy. Regular training improves the cardiorespiratory system's ability to maximally use oxygen. The largest amount of oxygen that you can consume per minute is called your maximal oxygen uptake. This maximal value, often referred to as your aerobic capacity, is a functional measure of your physical fitness. The maximum effort you can exert over a prolonged period of time is limited by your body's ability to deliver oxygen to the active tissues. Theoretically a higher oxygen uptake indicates an increased ability of the heart to pump oxygen-rich blood and of the muscle cells to use oxygen for energy production.

Regular vigorous exercise will produce a training effect that can increase your aerobic capacity by as much as 20 to 30 percent. **Aerobic capacity (VO_2max)** is the greatest amount of oxygen that you can consume per minute and is a functional measure of your physical fitness. The precise amount of increase depends on your pretraining status and on the intensity and duration of your training program. You might ask, why do I need a higher oxygen uptake? Maintaining an optimal aerobic capacity improves your energy levels for most activities and provides for a healthy cardiorespiratory system.

Maximal oxygen uptake gradually declines with age regardless of one's training status. Shortly after you reach adulthood (ages 18 to 21), your aerobic capacity begins to decline. However, the decrease is greater in inactive and overfat people and in those who have developed diseases of the heart and lungs.

Another training effect of cardiorespiratory exercise is the increased capacity of the exercising muscles to generate energy by using oxygen. Two key adaptations within muscle cells contribute to this improved capacity. First, there is an increase in the number, size, and membrane surface area of the mitochondria. Mitochondria are specialized compartments in the cells. These compartments contain the enzymes necessary for making the energy needed for muscular contraction. Thus mitochondria are the so-called powerhouses of the cells where energy is created. Second, training causes increases in the enzymes responsible for the creation of aerobic energy in muscles. In short, with increased numbers of powerhouses (mitochondria) and a corresponding increase in enzymes (compounds that accelerate the speed of chemical reactions), the trained muscle is able to produce greater amounts of energy and sustain higher levels of physical activity or performance.

Several studies have indicated that active people tend to have lower resting blood pressure rates than most sedentary people. Whether lowered blood pressure is a training effect of exercise alone is still questionable. If your blood pressure is normal, vigorous endurance-type exercise has little if any effect on your blood pressure. For people who already have serious health complications related to high blood pressure, the ability of exercise alone to lower blood pressure may be limited. However, the combination of an altered diet, medication, and exercise appears to be a promising approach to controlling this major risk factor for heart disease (see Chapter 11).

The evidence of the effects of exercise on the concentration levels of fat substances, or lipids, in the blood is encouraging. Cholesterol, triglycerides, and low-density and high-density lipoproteins are the blood lipids most often studied in heart disease research. This topic is discussed in greater detail in Chapter 11; for now, suffice it to say that people who are active and who adhere to sound nutritional practices tend to have a more favorable blood lipid profile, one that reduces their risk for heart disease.

Luckily the nonstop activities that benefit our heart and lungs also help us achieve and maintain ideal body composition by requiring steady amounts of energy. Many studies have shown that body fat can be reduced with regular vigorous training, particularly when combined with sensible eating. You may already notice that people who possess high levels of physical fitness are seldom overfat. A strong, lean physique is virtually impossible with dieting alone; a well-rounded exercise program is also necessary. Exercise plays a critical role not only in achieving but also in maintaining ideal body-fat levels throughout life.

The bones and muscles repetitively stressed during exercise benefit as well. Loss of bone mineral content (osteoporosis) is slowed or prevented, and muscular endurance is improved. And finally, although cardiorespiratory exercise improves physical fitness and health, most of these activities can also prepare people to participate in competitive sports.

Many people find cardiorespiratory endurance training to be uplifting and experience a mental high during and after a workout. Research studies have examined this cardiorespiratory exercise–induced increase in endorphins, substances produced in the pituitary gland, brain, and other tissues. These endorphins are said to have morphinelike qualities, reducing pain and producing a euphoric state. However, these studies have some limitations, and additional research is needed to fully comprehend the role of endorphins in producing this exercise-induced euphoria.

The next section discusses how to apply the four training specifics—type (mode), intensity, duration, and frequency—to cardiorespiratory endurance training. Proper application of these four factors will ensure an exercise program that is well within your present health and physical capabilities yet is geared toward your long-term goals. If you approach each of these four factors positively, you will see exercise as enjoyable, not as a dreaded task. For instance, instead of asking yourself, what type of exercise do I *have* to do?, ask yourself, what type of exercise do I *get* to do?

- *What type of exercise?* Continuous, rhythmic activities involving the large muscle groups
- *How hard?* 50 to 85 percent of heart-rate reserve
- *How long?* 20 to 60 minutes
- *How often?* Three to five days per week

Training Specifics

Mode: What Type of Exercise?

Exercises that utilize the large muscle groups and are rhythmic and continuous are recommended for improving and maintaining cardiorespiratory endurance. You may have heard this type of exercise called "aerobic exercise" because it involves the oxygen energy systems. These activities require large amounts of energy and are therefore also recommended for improving and maintaining ideal body composition. The intensity level of your chosen activity must be high enough to produce a training effect for your circulatory and respiratory systems. Because you can achieve a safe and reasonable intensity level by participating in a walking or a run-walk program, we recommend either for most beginners. However, if you have a low fitness level or any musculoskeletal problems, then we urge you to follow the guidelines suggested in the section on walking before doing any running.

It seems as if every few years, an exciting new type of cardiorespiratory exercise is introduced, attracting novices and experienced fitness enthusiasts alike. Many of these activities serve as alternatives to walking or running. The "menu" of cardiorespiratory activity choices today includes biking, swimming, rowing, dance aerobics, water aerobics, step aerobics, stair-stepping, cross-country skiing, rope skipping, sliding/lateral training, and in-line skating. Not only can these activities stand on their own as your chosen exercise mode, but two or more can be combined within the same workout for a cross-training program. As long as your exercise intensity stays in your target heart-rate range (more on this later) with continuous-type exertions, you can achieve your cardiorespiratory endurance goals. By cross-training, you add variety, which can improve your adherence to an exercise program. You also are able to utilize many different muscle groups, involving as many of your body's muscles as possible for balanced fitness.

Cardiorespiratory endurance activities can be categorized either as **weight-bearing exercise,** in which one or both feet maintain contact with the ground and support the body, or as **nonweight-bearing,** in which the exerciser is seated or buoyed up by water. Additionally cardiorespiratory exercise is categorized as either **nonimpact** (impact is not transferred from one foot to the other), **low-impact** (one foot always maintains contact with the exercise surface), **high-impact** (at some point both feet are off the exercise surface), or a combination of impacts. Choosing from different categories may minimize the chance for overuse injuries. Cardiorespiratory endurance activities other than walking or running are discussed in Chapter 6.

Never underestimate the role variety and convenience play in motivation and exercise adherence. Walking and running require no more equipment than a quality pair of shoes. But specialized cardiorespiratory exercise equipment—such as treadmills, stationary bicycles, rowing machines, ski machines, and stair-climbers—is also popular in fitness centers and in the home. Not only are these devices excellent sources of cardiorespiratory conditioning, but they add convenience and motivation to an exercise program. Videotapes for virtually all fitness activities are readily available for home use, and exercise machines frequently come with instructional videos as well.

When designing a fitness program, you should realize that low-intensity and short-duration activities produce low levels of improvement. In fact, they may not result in any fitness improvements. The relative values of various activities for improving physical fitness depend on the physiological intensity required. Thus golf, bowling, archery, and softball, to name a few sports, do little to develop or maintain cardiorespiratory endurance. These activities are great fun and may contribute to health maintenance, but they do not provide the necessary physiological stimulus and overload for developing or maintaining cardiorespiratory fitness. They simply do not require enough physical effort from your cardiorespiratory system.

If you have been inactive, you should avoid sprint-type fitness activities, which require sudden bursts of energy and quick movements. These types of activities are referred to as anaerobic (without oxygen). You first need to establish a good level of cardiorespiratory fitness, muscular strength and endurance, and flexibility. The older you grow, the more dangerous these activities become unless you are participating regularly in a physical fitness program. Keep in mind that in general, activities that require short bursts of speed and quick movements do little to improve your cardiorespiratory system unless integrated into a specific interval training program (see Chapter 9). Inclusion of these activities should be considered more for fun than for fitness.

Intensity: How Hard?

To improve cardiorespiratory endurance, a substantial overload is necessary. During exercise, the heart rate usually increases linearly with the energy requirement, as indicated by the amount of oxygen being used by the body (oxygen uptake). For this reason, the exercise heart rate represents a simple measure for estimating exercise intensity. Heart rate can be used to help you determine if you are exercising too hard or not hard enough to reach your fitness goals.

Many years ago, a study of young men yielded a minimum figure for the necessary increase in heart rate to achieve cardiorespiratory overload and subsequent improvement. M. J. Karvonen, a Finnish researcher, found that to make appreciable gains in cardiorespiratory endurance, the heart rate during exercise must be raised by approximately 60 percent of the difference between the resting and maximal heart rates. More recent research has led the American College of Sports Medicine to expand its guidelines for a **target heart-rate range.** Currently a safe and reasonable intensity for most participants ranges from 50 to 85 percent of the difference between resting and maximal rates. Calculating a target heart-rate range is simple. Take the difference between the maximal and resting rates, multiply it by 0.5 to 0.85, and add the result to the resting rate. This is called the 50- to 85-percent heart-rate reserve (HR reserve). In cases of overfatness or musculoskeletal limitations or after extended periods of inactivity, you may want to start out at 40- to 60-percent HR reserve.

An illustration using a 40-year-old man will make this calculation clear. His maximal heart rate can best be determined by a maximal graded exercise test, usually performed on a treadmill or bicycle ergometer. In the test, the man's work load is progressively increased, and his heart rate steadily increases along with the work load, until he reaches the point at which he can no longer continue the test. His heart rate at the point of maximal effort is considered his maximal heart rate. If a maximal graded exercise test is not available, his maximal heart rate will have to be approximated by subtracting his age from 220. (Although reasonably accurate, this predicted maximal heart rate can be off 10 to 12 beats in either direction. Keep this in mind if, in practice, your target heart-rate range seems slightly high or low.) This 40-year-old's approximate maximal heart rate would be 220 − 40 = 180 beats per minute. His resting heart rate, determined first thing upon waking, may be 80 beats per minute. His HR reserve is the difference between maximal and resting heart rates (180 − 80), or 100 beats. Fifty percent of 100 is 50 beats. Adding this figure to his resting rate of 80, we get a target heart rate of 130 beats per minute, a safe and reasonable lower end of the range for that individual. To find the upper end of his range, simply multiply HR reserve by 85 percent (100 × 0.85) and add that to his resting heart rate of 80. The highest heart rate in this 40-year-old's target heart-rate range, therefore, would be 165 beats per minute. The target heart-rate range represents intensities that are safe and, most important, effective in producing a training effect on the cardiorespiratory system. Figure 5.1 gives the simple formula for arriving at your target heart-rate range.

FIGURE 5.1
Target Heart-Rate Formula

Maximal heart rate (approximated) = 220 − your age _____

Resting heart rate = lowest of the day, taken upon waking _____

Lower end of the target heart-rate range = (max HR − resting HR) × 0.5 + resting HR _____

Upper end of the target heart-rate range = (max HR − resting HR) × 0.85 + resting HR _____

The value of this substantial overload in eliciting a training effect has been well documented. In general, for most young adults, this intensity means a target heart rate in the range of 150 to 170 beats per minute. For older adults, because of a typical decline in maximal heart rate with aging, a rate of 130 to 140 beats per minute may suffice. These intensities indicate safe and effective levels of vigorous exercise for healthy people.

Determining Your Heart Rate During Exercise

To determine your exercise intensity, you must find your pulse and count your heart rate during exercise, after you have broken a sweat or attained an intensity level you can describe as "moderately hard." It is perfectly acceptable to stop briefly to get a 10-second pulse count. Research reveals that this method gives a count indicative of your heart rate during exercise. Determining your heart rate relatively early in your workout lets you feel confident that you are in your target heart-rate range or signals you to adjust your intensity level either up or down. You will need a timing device such as a stopwatch, a wall clock, or a wristwatch with a second hand or digital readout.

Except in rare cases, the number of pulse beats you feel per minute is equal to your heart rate in beats per minute. Therefore your heart rate can be counted at any convenient pulse point. Generally the best places to check your pulse are on the carotid artery in your neck, on the radial artery on the inside of your wrist, or over your heart.

Taking your pulse at the radial artery may be your best option. To do so, place the tips of two fingers (not the thumb) on the inside of your wrist immediately below the base of the thumb. The carotid artery is located just under your jawbone, slightly behind your Adam's apple. Be sure to press lightly with fingers from the same side of your body as the carotid artery you choose. The heart pulse is on your chest, below and to the outside of your left nipple.

Whichever site you use, it is important to locate your pulse quickly. It will take a little practice, however, before you can consistently obtain a reliable pulse. In fact, you should first learn to count your resting pulse. Because your

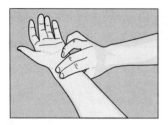 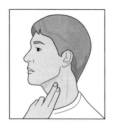 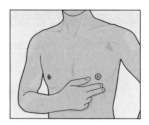

Three pulse locations

heart beats much slower at rest, counting the beats for 30 seconds and then multiplying by 2 gives the most accurate measure. During exercise, the heart rate declines rapidly if you stop moving, so it is important for you to learn to count your pulse as soon as possible (within a second or two after stopping).

When you feel your pulse, count the beats for 10 seconds beginning with 1. Then multiply your 10-second pulse count by 6 to determine your exercise heart rate in beats per minute. For example, a 10-second pulse count of 25 would indicate an exercise heart rate of 150 (25 × 6).

If for some reason you find it difficult to accurately count your pulse or are exercising without a timing device, you can use the rate of perceived exertion (RPE) to monitor your intensity level. By verbally describing how the exercise effort feels, you train yourself to get in touch with how hard you are working. For example, to reap cardiorespiratory endurance benefits, your exercise effort should rate as "moderately hard" to "hard" when you are working in your 60 to 80 percent target heart-rate range. Research shows that RPEs closely relate to actual exercise heart rate and provide a reliable guide to workout intensity. Nevertheless, we recommend that you become adept at locating your pulse to determine exercise heart rate. Then learn to associate your target heart rate with an overall feeling of adequate exertion. Down the road, you may find you don't need to check your pulse as often.

Duration: How Long?

The duration of exercise is directly related to the intensity of the activity, your present fitness level, and your fitness goals. Exertion at a 50- to 85-percent HR reserve enables you to spread a workout session over a longer period of time than is allowed at more intense levels of exercise. Training sessions of as little as 20 minutes in the target heart-rate range have been found to produce significant cardiorespiratory improvements. Our own experiences and research suggest that an exercise session of 30 minutes or longer is more likely to produce significant fitness changes. If you are beginning a program, however, you

---

WAY OF LIFE
Achieving a Proper Workout Intensity

- Fitness gains require some huffing and puffing, but not to the point of exhaustion.

- You should be able to rate your perceived exertion during cardiorespiratory exercise as being "moderately hard" to "hard."

- If you can carry on a conversation as you work out, you are working well within your capabilities. If you can easily sing, you may need to work a little harder.

- Counting your pulse during your workout allows you to adjust your intensity to make the most of your workout when it is needed.

- Prolonged fatigue for more than an hour after your workout is a sign that the exercise was too demanding.

- If your resting heart rate when you awake the day after a workout is five or more beats higher than normal, you may be overtraining and need to decrease workout intensity or duration or both until you recover.

---

should not try to continue for 30 minutes at a 50- to 85-percent HR reserve. To avoid musculoskeletal injuries, to allow your cardiorespiratory system to adjust to new demands, and to prepare yourself psychologically, begin with 20-minute sessions. An easy rule of thumb to follow concerning weekly increases in duration is the **10-percent program:** Increase your exercise duration by 10 percent each week to allow your body to adapt.

You can also incorporate "speedplay" at any level of fitness. Speedplay during an activity intersperses brief (30- to 60-second) recovery intervals of decreased intensity between your more vigorous segments at your target heart rate. These segments of milder exertion can occur whenever your body tells you to take a break. Continuing to move at a lesser intensity allows the metabolic waste products (such as lactic acid) in your bloodstream to be eliminated faster than they would be during complete rest. Continued contraction of your large muscles also guarantees that your blood will continue to circulate back to your heart from your extremities. Speedplay, with its intermittent recovery periods, allows you to extend your workout over a longer period of time. Furthermore, it ensures that your heart will pump rhythmically at a magnitude well above the resting rate throughout the complete workout. Specific workout plans for different cardiorespiratory activities will be discussed in Chapter 6.

Frequency: How Often?

Regular adherence to a vigorous program is necessary if you are to reach and maintain an adequate level of cardiorespiratory endurance. Don't count on limiting your exercise to physical education classes or weekend recreational activities. The number of workouts, or frequency, needed to achieve a cardiorespiratory training effect has been established by the American College of Sports Medicine at three to five sessions per week. Keep in mind that improvements in physical fitness require sustaining your workouts over 10 or more weeks. The first few weeks will be a break-in period. The recommended frequency of three to five days per week is based on the assumption that eventually your conditioning workouts will maintain an intensity of 50- to 85-percent HR reserve for a period of at least 20 minutes.

Your fitness workouts should be part of your life. Regular, purposeful exercise will provide you with abundant energy to make additional recreational activities enjoyable. Exercise regularity may also enable you to reach your fitness goals sooner, increasing your motivation. Although we have found that daily workouts are not necessary to improve one's cardiorespiratory endurance, they do tend to create a routine that becomes an essential part of your lifestyle. Daily workouts eliminate the possibility of dreading the workout days and relishing the "off" days.

Varying Exercise Mode, Intensity, Duration, and Frequency

Some people might do well to make slight adjustments to the regimen just presented when developing a personalized exercise program. Age, medical limitations, lifestyle, or excess body fat may make it necessary to vary the exercise mode, intensity, duration, and frequency components. For instance, some individuals might reduce intensity and use cross-training to decrease the chances for overuse injuries and psychological burnout resulting from daily workouts involving only one activity. In this case, if the intensity is less than the recommended 50- to 85-percent HR reserve, then the duration of the workout should be increased. Thus older people or people who are overfat or out of shape might start out with walking as their main exercise mode. Because walking involves a lower intensity of exercise than, say, running, a longer duration may be necessary.

Exercising to reduce body fat requires a different duration and frequency than exercising to improve cardiorespiratory endurance. To expend a significant amount of calories, you need to perform cardiorespiratory endurance activities five to seven days per week at a duration of 45 minutes or more. A controversy exists over the best time of day to exercise to reduce body fat.

Some research indicates that morning is optimal for using maximum amounts of fat for energy. Because the evidence is not conclusive, however, you should choose the time of day based on what fits your lifestyle. Plan to work out when you are feeling freshest, when you are least likely to make excuses not to exercise, and when the climate is optimal for you. Some people exercise in the evening before dinner because exercise suppresses their appetite to some extent. Others get too "keyed up" from nighttime exercise and find it difficult to fall asleep. If possible, remain flexible concerning your workout time so that if unusual circumstances arise, you can still fit your exercise session into your day.

The next section describes in detail walking and run-walk programs. These activities are the most common forms of cardiorespiratory endurance training and require only a good pair of shoes to get started. Chapter 6 will describe additional cardiorespiratory endurance activities.

Walking

Walking is a natural and beneficial form of cardiorespiratory exercise. It provides an adequate training stimulus as long as you maintain your target heart-rate range by walking at a quick pace or up an incline. You might decide to walk rather than run based on your fitness goals, preferences, and musculoskeletal injury profile. If you are trying to expend as much energy as possible in a given time period, running would be a better choice. A brisk 1-hour walk burns about 300 calories, whereas it takes only 30 minutes of running to burn the same amount or more. Because walking is low-impact (one foot is always in contact with the ground) and running is high-impact (both feet are off the ground at some point in the stride), walking is usually less stressful to joints than running. Walkers tend to have fewer injuries than runners, and for older people who have been very inactive over the years, walking is an excellent exercise choice. Regardless of age, if you are extremely overfat, walking is wiser than running until your body is better conditioned and you achieve a weight that your musculoskeletal system can safely support. If you have special medical limitations, such as bone or joint diseases, you may need to avoid running altogether. In these cases, walking as discussed in this chapter or any of the low-impact or nonimpact activities discussed in Chapter 6 may be the choice for you.

How to Walk for Fitness

A progressive program of walking using gradual increases in distance and intensity is one of the most suitable ways for some people to begin a fitness program. Walking for cardiorespiratory endurance is more than simply strolling with the dog. Even though you've been walking most of your life, fitness walking takes a little concentration at first. Begin walking at a comfortable, natural pace. Let your heel hit first and roll onto the ball of your foot. Push off with your toes. Maintaining a right-angle bend at your elbows, let your arms swing in a relaxed and rhythmic manner in opposition to your feet. Walk tall with your head high.

After a few walking sessions, your muscles and breathing will adjust to your pace. As you become comfortable, begin to pick up your pace. If it feels natural to lengthen your stride, extend your leg and foot farther in front and behind. Once you find a stride length that suits you, do not attempt to lengthen it to increase your speed. Instead, rely on moving your feet faster and pumping your arms more vigorously. Your hands can swing in an arc from your chest to your hip joint. Involve as many muscles as possible at a pace that constantly challenges your cardiorespiratory system. Strive to exercise in your target heart-rate range.

How to Start a Walking Program

After a 3- to 5-minute warm-up walking at a normal, easy gait, pick up your pace so that you maintain at least the lower end of your target heart-rate range. Check your pulse relatively early (around 5 minutes into your vigorous walk), after you begin sweating and can feel your heart and breathing rates elevate. Cover a mile if you can. If you do not have a measured route, try to walk nonstop for 15 minutes. As you become accustomed to the walking, try to increase the distance or duration by 10 percent per week until you can walk 2 miles or 30 minutes continuously. When you can accomplish 2 miles nonstop every day for a week, concentrate on increasing your walking speed to remain in your target heart-rate range. After you can walk 2 miles at a brisk pace in your target range, increase your distance or duration 10 percent per week to a daily 3 to 4 miles or 45 to 60 minutes. If you find it difficult to maintain a brisk steady pace, try speedplay. During speedplay, you periodically slow up for 30 to 60 seconds, and then return to your more intense pace until you feel the need to slow down again. But do not stop walking. Eventually you will be able to walk for 3 to 4 miles in 45 to 60 minutes. At this point, provided you have no joint injuries or any other health limitations, you may want to consider engaging in a run-walk or a running program.

If you plan to continue a walking program, you can achieve your training intensity in various ways. Carrying 1- to 3-pound weights in each hand while you walk has been a popular method of involving additional muscle groups. If you use these weights, make sure your arms and shoulders are sufficiently warmed up and that you maintain a bend in your elbows at all times. This additional energy expenditure may not add up to much unless you bring your hands to shoulder level on each forward arm pump.

To increase exercise intensity, you might also try a weighted hip belt, which is worn low over the hips and below the lower-back curve. Individual bars or pocket weights can be added progressively as you adjust to each new work load. Striding poles are another unique way of involving the large-muscle groups in the back, chest, and arms during a fitness walk. By reaching far forward and planting these rubber-tipped poles onto the ground, "pulling" your body by and then pushing behind you, you engage your upper body far more than during normal walking. Striding poles can be purchased at sporting goods stores, or you can make them yourself by wedging a tennis ball onto the point of a cross-country ski pole.

One method to avoid when trying to increase exercise intensity during walking is the use of ankle weights. Walking quickly with ankle weights turns your lower leg into a pendulum, the force of which can place excessive strain on the knees, hips, and back. Save the ankle weights for muscular strength exercises.

Run-Walk: A Basic Program

Minute for minute, running is one of the most effective cardiorespiratory and energy-expending activities. Running is such a simple activity in which to participate. The only "equipment" you need is shock-absorbant shoes. Most important, you can run any time that is convenient in your busy schedule. Even bad weather should not hold you back, provided you dress properly and take the necessary precautions.

The run-walk technique of conditioning can be used all by itself as a highly effective cardiorespiratory activity or as a stepping-stone for beginning a running program. In either case, the approach presented here is based on more than three decades of successful programs with schoolchildren, college

---

WAY OF LIFE
Facts About Walking and Running (for a 150-pound person)

- Walking uses about 5 calories per minute, so walking a 20-minute mile consumes about 100 calories.

- Running uses about 10 calories per minute, so running a 10-minute mile consumes about 100 calories.

- Shoes worn for walking or running tend to break down after approximately 400 miles and should be replaced at this point.

- Walking is the most popular fitness activity engaged in by adults in America.

students, and adults. Its fundamental strength is the ease with which individual needs can be met, regardless of age or level of physical fitness.

How to Run for Fitness

The skill of running is often taken for granted. Frequently the beginning runner starts plodding around a track or down a street without any instruction and wonders why it doesn't feel right. The repetitive cadence of an experienced runner looks simple and natural. The smooth interaction of the parts of the body while running represents an efficiency of movement for which there is no magic formula. However, certain practices can help you improve your running technique.

Proper posture while running is essential for good body mechanics. Good posture requires muscular strength and endurance (discussed in detail in Chapter 7). People with poor muscular strength and mechanics tend to let their abdomens sag, they lean too far forward with their chests and heads, and they run with their buttocks projecting behind them. Such a posture hampers a smooth and efficient running style and can also produce lower-back pain. With good running posture, you keep your spine straight, your head up, your shoulders and hips level, and your elbows bent approximately at right angles. Your arm swing and running stride should feel comfortable and relaxed. As you moves your body may lean slightly in the direction you are running.

It's important not to run on your toes. Many beginning runners start this way and quickly learn this technique is appropriate only when sprinting a short distance. The flatfoot or the heel-to-the-ball-of-the-foot landing are the accepted techniques in fitness running. These methods place the maximum amount of shoe surface on the ground with each landing. In the flatfoot landing, the sole of the foot lands squarely on the ground. The heel (rear-foot) landing is quite similar except that you set your heel down first, roll your weight along the sole, and push off with the ball of your foot and your toes. In other words, you run almost flat-footed, with your heel touching the ground slightly before the ball of your foot. In both methods, the foot should touch the ground as lightly as possible. A little practice will help you develop a smooth and efficient rhythm.

Overstriding is another common mistake made by many inexperienced runners. Overstriding results in the lead foot striking the ground too far ahead of your body, causing a jerky, inefficient motion. There is an optimal stride length for you. Experiment to find one that allows you to cover a good distance with each step without forcing your hip, knee, and ankle joints to go beyond their comfortable range of motion.

Other common faults include running with toes pointing inward or outward, bouncing excessively, carrying arms and hands too high (above the shoulders), and swinging the hands across the center line of the body. Strive to run as smoothly as possible, eliminating all excess movements.

Regulating Run-Walking and Running Intensity

Running is defined here as moving at a pace that covers over 220 yards (half the distance around a regulation outdoor quarter-mile track) in 60 to 90 seconds. This is equivalent to running an 8- to 12-minute mile. This pace, we have found, is well within the capability of most people starting a running program. Keep in mind that you do not have to run at a punishing pace to provide an adequate stimulus to your cardiorespiratory system. At first, runs of 110 to 220 yards (100 to 200 meters) are recommended, followed by 30-second periods of brisk walking. These run-walk combinations are repeated throughout the workout. The walking segments are an important part of this rhythmic routine because they represent a semirecovery period. However, the heart rate must remain in the target range regardless of whether you walk or run.

If you do not have access to a measured track, running for specific time segments such as 30 seconds, 60 seconds, or longer followed by periods of brisk walking can produce a similar training stimulus. An easy way to progress to more running and less walking is to use 60 seconds as a unit that is repeated throughout a workout (keep in mind that you should strive to keep moving for 20 minutes). In stage 1, run for 15 seconds and then walk for 45 seconds. When comfortable, progress to stage 2, running and walking for 30 seconds each. In stage 3, run for 45 seconds and then walk for 15 seconds. Finally, in stage 4, run for at least 60 seconds or more. If you need to slow down to a walk, retreat to stage 3. Eventually walking will constitute little, if any, of your workout.

The most common mistake when starting a run-walk program is to run too fast. The key to a truly individualized program is to establish your own running pace. Adjust this pace by checking your pulse frequently, slowing down or speeding up to stay at approximately 50- to 85-percent HR reserve. Remember, don't wait until your run is over to find out you exercised too hard or not hard enough. Your perceived exertion should be "moderately hard" to "hard." Regulate your workout by increasing or reducing your speed (pace) or the number of run-walk bouts, or sets (see Table 5.1).

The Run-Walk Workout

We have just discussed general approaches to a run-walk program; now let's look at specific progressive steps for starting one. You can choose to run either for a certain period of time or for a predetermined distance. Table 5.1 is organized in steps so that you can gradually increase the distance or the time of your runs (maintaining the same speed) until you can cover a mile or more continuously. Being able to run 2 miles or for 15 to 20 minutes represents a minimal goal for most men and women. Ultimately your goal is to sustain running for 30 minutes per session or for a distance of 3 to 4 miles or more. These steps are especially suitable for young people possessing good health.

TABLE 5.1
Run-Walk Workout

Step	Run*	Walk	Load	Approximate Distance Covered
1	Run 110 yd (30 – 45 sec.).	Walk 30 sec.	Start with 8 sets*; in each succeeding workout, try to add a set until you can complete 12 sets; then go on to the next step.	1/2 – 3/4 mile
2	Run 220 yd (1 – 1.5 min.).	Walk 30 sec.	Start with 6 sets; in each succeeding workout, try to add a set until you can complete 12 sets; then go on to the next step.	3/4 – 1 1/2 miles
3	Run 440 yd (2 – 3 min.).	Walk 30 – 45 sec.	Start with 6 sets; in each succeeding workout, try to add a set until you can complete 10 sets; then go on to the next step.	1 1/2 – 2 1/2 miles
4	Run 880 yd (4 – 6 min.).	Walk 30 – 45 sec.	Start with 4 sets; in each succeeding workout, try to add a set until you can complete 6 sets in succession for two days; then go on to the next step.	2 – 3 miles
5	Run 1 mile (8 – 12 min.).	Walk 1 – 2 min.	Start with 2 sets; in each succeeding workout, try to add a set until you can complete 4 sets (4 one-mile runs); then go on to the next step.	2 – 4 miles
6	Run 1 1/2 miles (12 – 16 min.).	Walk 2 – 3 min.	After you run the first 1 1/2 miles and walk, try to run another 1 1/2 miles, or run only 880-yd. segments alternated with walking. When you are able to run a second 1 1/2 miles continuously, go to the next step, continuous running.	3 miles or more
7	Continuous running: run 2 – 4 miles.	Cool down: walk 5 min. or more.	—	2 – 4 miles

* A set represents one run-walk bout.

Table 5.1 specifies the load (exercise work load) recommended for each step in terms of sets. One set combines a run and the ensuing walk. Gradually increasing the number of sets increases the work load that produces the training effect. This initial conservative approach will prevent unnecessary injury or soreness, which could terminate the entire fitness program. Also, your running segments will be at a faster tempo than they would be if you struggled along for 10 minutes or so without stopping. These shorter but faster runs will effectively lead to longer-duration, nonstop running. You may wish to stay with a specific work load for each step (number of sets) for two workouts before adding another set. Remember, when you recover fully and do not feel overly fatigued an hour after a workout, you are ready to move up to the next work load within that step.

Both running and walking segments are performed anywhere in your target heart-rate range at a perceived exertion of "moderately hard" to "hard." To make sure you are working within your own capacity, try the "talk test" while you're running. If you cannot carry on a conversation without becoming short of breath, then you're probably overexerting.

If you evaluated your cardiorespiratory endurance with the 1.5-mile running test (see Chapter 3), your results can help you determine a suitable starting point. If you scored in the "poor" category, begin with step 1; if you scored in the "fair" or "average" category, try step 2; if you scored in the "good" category, start with step 2 (10 sets) or possibly step 3; and if you scored in the "excellent" category, you can begin anywhere from step 3 through step 7. At this level of cardiorespiratory endurance, the step you choose for starting your workout depends on your previous running experience. If you are in good shape but have not been running on a regular basis, then start at step 3, 4, or 5. However, if you already run regularly, then you probably don't need the table. In that case, however, you could use the run-walk routine as an interval training program to improve your time (see Chapter 9). One suggestion for those coming from the walking program and starting with step 1: Walk briskly for 8 to 10 minutes prior to your running sets. Follow up your prescribed run-walk repeats with another 6 to 8 minutes of brisk walking. This helps make the transition from walking to running less traumatic at the outset and helps avoid injury. In fact, a few minutes of brisk walking before any running is recommended.

Summary

A sound cardiorespiratory endurance program is geared to your individual capabilities and needs and adequately stimulates your heart, lungs, and muscles. Whether you develop a walking, run-walking, or running program, it is important to sustain a target heart rate well above the resting rate but not at an exhaustive level. As you progress in your conditioning, you will be able to do more exercise at the same target heart rate; that is, you will be walking or running faster, but you won't feel as if you are trying any harder. Thus, if your heart rate is 162 while running at a 10-minute-per-mile pace at the start of a program, after three months of training you may be able to run an $8\frac{1}{2}$-minute-per-mile pace at the same heart rate. The bonus is that you will be using more energy at the faster tempo, expending more calories per workout. The programs suggested in this chapter can easily be modified to suit your individual needs.

After you begin to notice some improvement, you may wish to retest yourself on the cardiorespiratory endurance tests in Chapter 3. For example, the time it takes you to run 1.5 miles following a 6- to 8-week run-walk or running program can give you some indication of your improvement in cardiorespiratory endurance. Remember, you can always improve and set new goals with a variety of activities throughout your life!

Key Words

AEROBIC CAPACITY/VO$_2$MAX: The greatest amount of oxygen that you can consume per minute; a functional measure of your physical fitness.

HIGH-IMPACT EXERCISE: Endurance activities in which both feet are off the exercise surface at one point or another.

LOW-IMPACT EXERCISE: Endurance activities in which one foot always maintains contact with the exercise surface.

NONIMPACT EXERCISE: Endurance activities without an air-borne phase, in which the exerciser is seated or buoyed by water.

NONWEIGHT-BEARING EXERCISE: Endurance activities in which the exerciser is seated or buoyed up by water.

TARGET HEART-RATE RANGE: The range in heart rate necessary to achieve cardiorespiratory overload and subsequent improvement in cardiorespiratory endurance; 50 to 85 percent of heart-rate reserve, according to the American College of Sports Medicine.

10-PERCENT PROGRAM: An easy and safe rule of thumb to follow concerning weekly increases in duration in cardiorespiratory endurance training.

TRAINING EFFECT: Gradual improvements to the exercised heart, lungs, and muscles that allow them to function at a higher level both during physical exertion and at rest.

WEIGHT-BEARING EXERCISE: Endurance activities in which one or both feet maintain contact with the ground and support the body.

A Way of Life Library

Brown, R. L., and J. Henderson. *Fitness Running.* Champaign, IL: Human Kinetics, 1994.

Cooper, K. H. *The Aerobics Program for Total Well-Being.* New York: Bantam Books, 1982.

Fixx, J. F. *The Complete Book of Running.* New York: Random House, 1977.

Noakes, T. D. *Lore of Running.* Champaign, IL: Human Kinetics, 1991.

Seaborg, E., and E. Dudley. *Hiking and Backpacking.* Champaign, IL: Human Kinetics, 1994.

Sheehan, G. *Dr. Sheehan on Running.* Mountain View, CA: World Publications, 1975.

CHAPTER 6

Cardiorespiratory Endurance Activities

This chapter describes in detail the various cardiorespiratory activities aside from walking and running that you can choose for your personal exercise program. Each activity offers something unique. We highly recommend that you try as many activities as possible and consider using more than one to achieve your own fitness goals.

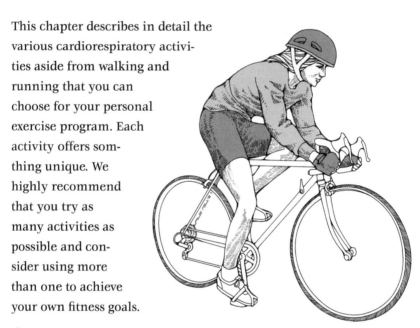

As you read this chapter, keep these statements in mind:

- The best cardiorespiratory endurance activity for you is the one that you enjoy most and that best fits your lifestyle.
- The key to a personalized program is to establish your own exercise pace based on your heart-rate response to your workout.
- As a general rule, you must cycle almost twice as fast as you would run to produce the same training heart rate.
- Swimming is an excellent nonimpact conditioner, and even a relatively unskilled swimmer can get an adequate workout in the water.
- Indoor cardiorespiratory equipment such as the treadmill, stationary bike, rowing machine, stair-climber, and cross-country skier, as well as various forms of aerobic activity, are also very effective in providing a total-body stimulus.

Bicycling

Cycling workouts based on physiological training principles not only can enhance your cardiorespiratory endurance but also can be very pleasurable. Bike rides, whether as family get-togethers or in outings with friends, can provide camaraderie and a good excuse to be outdoors. Bicycling is also an excellent nonimpact alternative to running.

Bicycling for cardiorespiratory endurance requires vigorous, sustained pedaling in your target heart-rate range for 20 to 60 minutes to stimulate your lungs, heart, and muscles adequately. Racing requires an even higher level of physical fitness, and many hours of riding and other forms of conditioning are necessary if you want to ride competitively. Naturally the speed at which you ride, just as in walking and running, will determine your cycling intensity. In general, riding at a pace of 4 to 6 minutes per mile (10 to 15 mph) is equivalent to a 50- to 85-percent HR reserve intensity for most people.

Safety Considerations

Frankly it takes some skill and savvy to ride a bicycle effectively, especially one with many gears. You must learn to operate your bicycle in an efficient and safe manner. This means being able to control your bike under all conditions. You should be able to brake properly, turn corners, and navigate tight situations such as narrow pathways and traffic.

More than a million people a year are injured in bicycle accidents, and roughly 1,000 of them die. Many of these accidents are caused by faulty equipment and poor cycling techniques. In an effort to reduce the number of bicycle accidents, the U.S. Consumer Product Safety Commission has set rigid safety standards for all bicycles marketed today. Thus your first need is a bike in good working condition that meets the commission's standards. Before embarking on a cycling training program, allow yourself adequate practice time to become familiar with the brakes, gear shifting, and high-speed riding. These "bike basics" may be best practiced on a bike trail. Also check that the tires are inflated properly (the recommendations usually are imprinted on the tire itself). The self-confidence you develop from knowing your equipment will help you to meet emergency situations without panic. Many colleges, YMCAs, and adult education programs offer classes in bicycling that also include mechanical care and repair of your bike. Such courses are highly recommended.

Cycling also requires an awareness of the actions of other users of the road and a realization of your limitations and those of your equipment. Until you are an experienced cyclist, avoid heavy traffic, steep and winding roads, and long-distance rides. Because you are considered a vehicle when on a bike, you must ride on the right-hand side of public roads. Also, use hand signals to indicate turns and stops, and obey traffic signals as if you were driving an automobile. If riding with other cyclists, make sure you ride single file.

Equipment and Clothing

If you want to cycle regularly, find a reputable bike shop to assist and advise you in choosing and maintaining your equipment. Your bike will need periodic checkups and brake, steering, and gear adjustments. Unless you are quite handy, a good mechanic is a must. A qualified professional will help you choose either a mountain bike (wider tires), a road/racing bike (thinner tires), or a hybrid of the two, depending on where and how you intend to ride. Regardless of the type of bike you ride, an odometer and time clock should be standard equipment for checking heart rate and pace per mile.

After you have selected your bike, adjust the seat to the proper height for you. Many people ride with the seat too low, placing undue strain on their knee joints. When you are sitting on the seat with the balls of your feet on the pedals, your knee joints should be slightly bent when each pedal is at its lowest point. This alignment places the large thigh muscles in the most advantageous position when you pedal with the ball of the foot. Toe clips allow you not only to use the hip and knee extensor muscles to push the pedal downward but also to engage the flexor muscles to help pull the pedal back up again. More recent innovations also include streamlined handlebars that allow you to rest your elbows on pads while lowering your trunk into a more aerodynamic position.

A helmet is a must. Even those of us with "hard heads" can't compete with a road! You reduce your risk of a head injury by 85 percent and your risk of a brain injury by almost 90 percent when you wear a helmet. Many cyclists who have fallen have been saved from serious injury (and even death) because they wore protective headgear. The cost of a well-made helmet is a small price to pay for the injury protection it offers. The bulky helmets of the past have been replaced with a host of cool, colorful, and sleek models. These helmets are more aerodynamic and much lighter than previous models. Before you consider color, fashion, or price, however, look inside for a sticker indicating that the helmet has been certified by the American National Standards Institute (ANSI) or the Snell Memorial Foundation. The Snell standard is considered to be more stringent. The Bicycle Federation of America states that consumers can be confident of the safety and durability of a helmet as long as it bears one of the safety stickers and is made by a reputable company.

For serious cycling workouts, street clothes are too confining for efficient and enjoyable training. Today clothing specifically designed to maximize comfort and mobility is readily available. Bicycle wear is lightweight, streamlined, unrestricting, durable, and, most important, protective. Cycling shorts should be long enough to keep the skin on your legs from rubbing against the saddle. The seams should be flat to avoid abrasion. Sewn into the seat and crotch area

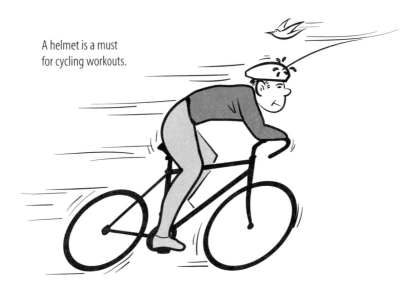

A helmet is a must
for cycling workouts.

of your shorts should be a large piece of chamois (soft leather) that reduces friction between you and the saddle. Regardless of your clothing choice, wear bright colors that contrast with your surroundings so that you are highly visible to motorists. Cycling gloves provide padding to reduce pressure points on your hands, and they keep sweat from creating a slippery grip. Many people ride in running or cross-training shoes, which are adequate for most fitness cyclists. The serious cyclist uses special shoes with a stiff sole and cleat, but these are probably not necessary at the outset of your cycling program.

Finding a Place to Train

Because cycling for cardiorespiratory endurance requires nonstop vigorous pedaling, the inevitable starts and stops associated with city streets rule them out as the best riding paths. Country roads tend to provide safer workouts. In fact, if these roads are within a 10-minute ride, many cyclists use the slower city-street riding as their warm-up. By the time they reach the less-traveled roads, their heart rates have reached their target ranges. Regional bicycling associations or clubs frequently organize touring rides and know all the "secret routes" that provide the best roadways in your area. Check with local bike shops or the phone book for these organizations.

Forest preserves, nature parks, and other public recreational facilities provide designated bike paths and trails. Unless these trails are restricted to bike use only, be certain to watch for hikers or runners. Many cities and towns are developing biking trails along old railway lines in "Rails to Trails" programs. Check with your local parks and recreation department for locations near you.

Snow and hard rain are obvious deterrents to a good cardiorespiratory workout on a bike. One option for cyclists who prefer their outdoor bike to an indoor stationary cycle is to invest in a "spin trainer." Cyclists mount their outdoor bike on this type of bike stand, which keeps the wheels from contacting the floor during temporary indoor use.

Training with a Bicycle

To achieve a training effect with a bicycle, you need to pedal vigorously enough to stress the heart and lungs sufficiently. You must cycle almost twice as fast as you would run in order to produce the same exercise heart rate.

For those of you who have not been active in recent months, your first few weeks of riding will be at relatively low speeds with a gradual buildup of total distance each session. You want to reach the point at which you can sustain a continuous ride for at least 15 minutes. At this point, you are ready to begin a more vigorous regimen (see Table 6.1). Your goal is to train your cardiorespiratory system so that you can steadily pump your legs at a perceived exertion of "moderately hard" to "hard" for 40 to 60 minutes.

The Workout

Intermittent activity similar to the run-walk format, using either distance repeats or timed repeats, is a simple approach for conditioning with a bicycle. Distance repeats require cycling a preselected distance (such as a quarter mile, half mile, or perhaps even a mile) at a tempo ranging from 10 to 20 miles per hour. Your own cycling tempo depends on your fitness and, of course, on your heart-rate response to the cycling work. After each vigorous distance ride, continue cycling at a slower tempo (but still in your target heart-rate range) for between 30 seconds and 2 minutes. This recovery period of slow cycling is analogous to the walking portion of a run-walk session, and you should maintain your target heart-rate range throughout the conditioning segment. When you complete this recovery period, resume the faster cycling tempo for the preselected distance. When you ride short distances (a quarter mile or half mile), your recovery rides should be relatively short (30 to 45 seconds). When you ride longer distances (1 or 2 miles), your recovery rides should be lengthened accordingly.

An example of timed repeats would be vigorous cycling for a 2- to 4-minute period (or, in fact, for any time period for which you can endure and maintain the target heart-rate range). Follow this more intense exercise with a recovery period at a reduced pedaling speed. Then repeat the process.

If you gauge your work load properly, either distance repeats or timed repeats will give you sufficient exercise during a 30- to 45-minute session. And there are many possible variations in these routines. Although it is impractical

| | | | | Approximate |
Step	Vigorous Cycling*	Slow Cycling	Load	Distance Covered
1	1 mile or 5 min. (12 mph).	$1/4$ mile or 2 min.	Start with 5 sets; in each succeeding workout, add a set until you can do 8 sets.	5 – 8 miles
2	1 mile or 4 min. (15 mph).	$1/4$ mile or 2 min.	Start with 5 sets; in each succeeding workout, add a set until you can do 10 sets.	5 – 10 miles
3	$1^1/_2$ miles or 6 min. (15 mph).	$1/3$ mile or 3 min.	Start with 4 sets; in each succeeding workout, add a set until you can do 10 sets.	6 – 15 miles
4	2 miles or 8 min. (15 mph).	$1/3$ mile or 3 min.	Start with 4 sets; in each succeeding workout, add a set until you can do 10 sets.	8 – 20 miles
5	10 – 20 miles or 40 min. to $1^2/_3$ hrs. of continuous cycling (12 – 15 mph).	Every 5 miles, you may wish to cycle for a mile at a reduced speed.	—	10 – 20 miles

TABLE 6.1 Bicycling Repeats

*The cycling speed needs to provide a heart-rate stimulus of 50- to 85-percent HR reserve; the speed suggested may have to be altered to meet your particular training needs.

to present them all here, Table 6.1 shows a beginning sequence of workouts with a bicycle for a young adult.

After you try the workout in Table 6.1, you may need to adjust the intensity (cycling speed) to provide a lesser or greater heart-rate stimulus. Once you become accustomed to your cycling workouts, you can devise many other workout variations that will be appropriate to your interests and needs. You may even decide to do a long-distance touring trip (50 to 100 miles a day) during a vacation or on a weekend. Whether you tour or perform a series of timed repeats of fast and slow cycling, you will find the bicycle an excellent device for developing and maintaining cardiorespiratory endurance.

Swimming

Swimming is another excellent means of developing cardiorespiratory endurance. Not only is it one of the most enjoyable forms of exercise, it is a superb choice for people who are unable to participate in weight-bearing activities. The rhythmic movement of the upper-body muscles in particular also make swimming an excellent cross-training choice to couple with walking, running, and cycling for total body involvement. Besides, the stimulation of the cool water is refreshing.

Because swimming offers five basic strokes to choose from, combining two or more strokes within a workout can minimize the chance of suffering overuse injuries. A simple variation of strokes not only gives an abbreviated rest for some specific muscles but allows other muscle groups to be actively exercised and stimulated.

Swimming does have certain drawbacks. For one thing, you must know how to swim! If you cannot, we suggest that you take advantage of the opportunities to learn to swim in your community or school. No one should graduate from college without learning to swim, particularly from a safety standpoint. If you already know the basics, take advantage of any opportunities to brush up on your technique. Videotapes offering expert advice and demonstrations on stroke mechanics are available at sporting goods stores or through sports equipment catalogs. By improving your swimming skills, you gain confidence around water and can concentrate on improving your endurance rather than simply trying to stay afloat. For those with an inclination towards competitiveness, organized swim teams offer fun, vigorous workouts and meets with other swimmers of all ages.

One additional drawback to swimming for fitness is not having regular access to a pool. Being able to swim without interruptions in an open lane is a necessity. Recently more and more pools across the country are setting aside designated times for lap swimming. Home pools that are too short to enable good lap swimming can be adapted for tethered swimming. A simple piece of rubberized tubing with one end attached to a swimmer's ankle or waist and the other end to any immovable object on the perimeter of the pool (such as a ladder or diving board stand) can provide just enough stretch and resistance to swim in place. You can also pack this tubing into a suitcase and use it in a hotel pool when on business trips or vacations.

Equipment and Clothing

Swimsuits for fitness swimming can be of any material as long as they are comfortable. Competitive racing suits are usually a lycra or nylon blend, making them sleek and drag-resistant. However, to increase workout intensity, some swimmers purposely increase water drag by wearing multiple suits or even mesh swim vests with pockets that catch the water as the swimmer moves forward.

It's best to wear swim goggles to protect your eyes from irritation due to pool water chemicals. Goggles come in different sizes and shapes to fit various eye sockets. Try the suction test when looking for swim goggles. Without the strap around your head, lightly press the eye pieces into a comfortable position on your eye sockets. If the goggles stay put for a brief time, they fit correctly and will maintain the seal around your eyes when swimming.

A small digital clock can be adhered to the upper corner of swim goggles to monitor swim pace and workout times without your having to stop and check a wristwatch. Also, to keep track of your heart rate, you can purchase a waterproof heart rate monitor similar to those worn on land.

More advanced swimmers also use hand paddles, kick boards, and swim fins to sharpen their "feel" for the water and to adjust their body position in the water. It is important not to warm up with these aids, because they overexaggerate limb movements and may irritate the joints. It is also not a good idea to use them as a crutch to compensate for poor technique.

Swim Training

The five basic swim strokes are the sidestroke, breaststroke, front crawl (freestyle), backstroke, and butterfly. The last four are the competitive strokes. The sidestroke and breaststroke typically are the slowest and require the least amount of energy because arms are not lifted out of the water. The front crawl is the fastest stroke and would therefore be the stroke of choice when you are trying to maximize your workout distance in a given time. However, frontcrawl kicking is not highly taxing on the leg muscles because its main function is to keep the body horizontal in the water. The backstroke involves more leg muscle involvement and gives swimmers a chance to enjoy the sunshine (and a change of scenery) during a workout. The butterfly requires both arms to leave the water at once and therefore is the most strenuous of the five strokes. Swimming a few lengths of "fly" (a length equals 25 yards) would certainly elevate a sluggish heart rate into the target range (and maybe beyond).

If you are a good swimmer, we recommend continuous swimming. To vary the workout, you can swim a different stroke every four lengths. Changing strokes systematically (such as four lengths of freestyle, four lengths of backstroke, and four lengths of breaststroke) makes it easier to keep track of the number of lengths completed. Again, if the intensity is vigorous enough, a minimum of 20 minutes in the water per session will provide a physically profitable and refreshing experience. A simple way to keep track of your lengths completed is to keep a pile of pennies on the pool deck to the left side of your lane. Each time you finish four lengths, move a penny to the right side. If you predetermine how many lengths you wish to swim, start with one-fourth that amount of pennies. When the penny pile is depleted, your workout is over.

The Workout

Even a relatively unskilled swimmer can carry out a productive cardiorespiratory endurance workout. The only requirement is that you be able to swim at

TABLE 6.2
Swimming Repeats

Step	Swim*	Walk†	Load	Approximate Distance Covered
1	Swim 1 length (30 – 40 sec.).	Get out of the pool and walk back to the starting point (30 sec.).	Start with 10 sets; in each succeeding workout, try to add 2 sets until you reach 20 sets.	250 – 500 yd
2	Swim 2 lengths (60 – 80 sec.).	Get out of the pool and walk to the other end of the pool (30 sec.).	Start with 8 sets; in each succeeding workout, try to add 2 sets until you reach 20 sets.	400 – 1,000 yd
3	Swim 3 lengths (90 – 120 sec.).	Get out of the pool and walk back to the starting point (45 sec.).	Start with 6 sets; in each succeeding workout, try to add 2 sets until you reach 15 sets.	450 – 1,125 yd
4	Swim 4 lengths (120 – 160 sec.).	Get out of the pool and walk to the other end of the pool (60 sec.).	Start with 4 sets; in each succeeding workout, try to add 2 sets until you reach 16 sets.	400 – 1,600 yd

*One length is equal to 25 yards.

† In some situations, it may not be possible to get out of the pool and walk; thus you may have to rest for 30 seconds or more in the water at the end of the pool.

least one length of the pool. A simple workout is to swim one length of the pool, then climb out and walk back to the other end of the pool where you started. Repeat this procedure. In some situations, it may not be possible to get out of the pool to walk. Instead, you may choose to rest in the water at the end of the pool. Moderate movements of your legs as you rest will aid your recovery between vigorous swims. Or, if the pool is shallow enough, you can walk in the water, which has the added benefit of water resistance to keep your heart rate in the target range. This swim-walk routine is similar to the running and cycling techniques we have already described. Later on, you can increase the intensity of the work load by swimming two lengths in succession before walking a length or resting at the end of the pool. Remember, switching strokes offers the benefit of continuous movement while allowing certain muscle groups a slight rest.

Table 6.2 provides a sequence of workouts for beginning a swimming fitness program. In this series of swims, it is assumed that you will periodically check your heart rate to ensure that you are working in the 50- to 85-percent

HR reserve level. It is well documented that when you are prone (lying face down in the water), your heart rate is anywhere from 8 to 12 beats lower than when you exercise upright. If you swim with a heart-rate monitor, you can check this yourself. Keep this in mind and don't get frustrated if you fall short of your usual land-based target range. Determine your special swimming target range and rely on perceived exertion, swimming at an intensity of "moderately hard" to "hard."

Once you achieve step 4 of the swim program, you have many options. If you have good swimming skills, you can swim continuously for $\frac{1}{2}$ to 1 mile (approximately 900 to 1,800 yards). In general, 100 yards of swimming equals about 400 yards of running; thus a half mile of swimming is equivalent to about 2 miles of running.

Aerobics/Aerobic Dance

Since the late 1960s and early 1970s, aerobic dance, or **aerobics,** has been a very popular form of exercise. The term *aerobic* literally means "with oxygen." However, most people connect aerobics with exercise involving vigorous movements performed to music. Along with more complex dance-oriented routines, aerobics instructors lead workouts involving walking, running, hopping, skipping, kicking, and various arm swings. Aerobics classes can be accompanied by virtually any type of music.

A properly planned aerobics class offers a good cardiorespiratory workout using most muscles of the body and requiring large amounts of energy. Studies have shown that the energy requirements of aerobics workouts can range from 4 to 10 calories or more per minute, depending on the movements and tempo. Classes also typically include exercises to develop flexibility, strength, and muscular endurance. And the release of emotional and mental tension through self-expression to music is an added bonus.

Aerobics can take the form of aerobic dance, high-impact, low-impact, or high/low-impact aerobics. Classes may combine two or more of these forms within the same workout. Aerobic dance consists of choreographed routines that typically repeat movements when phrases in the music repeat. The routines remain the same from workout to workout, which builds confidence and frees participants to enjoy the movements without requiring too much concentration. One drawback is the necessity to stop and learn each new routine at its introduction. This makes it difficult to maintain the target heart-rate range.

High-impact, low-impact, or combination high/low-impact aerobics are more free-form, taking shape from movements the instructor mixes and matches depending on the class response. **High-impact aerobics** are so-called because the body is propelled off the floor and both feet are off the ground at the same time. Because the resulting forceful landings place stress on the feet and lower legs, participants and instructors are at risk for injury. Thus **low-impact aerobics** evolved, in which one foot is always in contact with the floor. Studies have shown that low-impact aerobics can provide a cardiorespiratory stimulus, especially if the body is kept lower to the ground to use the large muscle groups of the thighs and buttocks. Arm movements also need to be kept at least at shoulder height to elevate the heart rate. Because some individuals enjoy both impact levels and do not suffer from impact-induced injuries, a combination using both high- and low-impact moves is a very popular choice for classes of varying fitness and age levels. The key to any of these forms is to keep moving continuously throughout the workout.

As in running and walking, quality shoes are the only equipment needed to participate in aerobics. Aerobics shoes differ from running shoes in that they provide more shock absorption at the balls and arches of the feet, where landing takes place. There is also no "waffling" or nubs on the soles, because twisting and lateral sliding movements are typical. Just as important as your shoe is the surface on which you perform aerobics. Never exercise on concrete or linoleum, and stay away from carpet if possible (it is easy to snag your foot on the carpet nap). Wooden floors are preferable, particularly floors suspended over air space or additional shock-absorbant materials. If you perform aerobics at home, at least have some kind of shock-reducing material such as a nonskid exercise mat under your feet to reduce the risk of impact injuries.

Some aerobics exercisers work out with 1- to 3-pound hand weights. The purpose of these weights is to assist in elevating the heart rate and burning additional calories. Just as in walking, these weights must be lifted at least to shoulder height to significantly raise the energy requirement. Controlled motions are imperative, and you must maintain correct posture and not overload the shoulder or elbow joints. It's also important to attend to the safety of the other exercisers around you. Before attempting to use outside resistance to increase exercise intensity, many exercisers find that by simply paying more attention to correct form, especially with low-impact aerobics, they can increase intensity to the desired level.

The key to the popularity of aerobics is that it is fun and offers variety. Many people wouldn't be exercising today if they hadn't started out with aerobics. Another attraction of aerobics is group involvement with a leader. But having to attend a regular class can also be a drawback. For people who want to do their own thing in the privacy of their homes, a plethora of videotapes can be purchased or rented. Unfortunately many of these tapes include activities that have the potential for injury. Because exercise videotapes are so popular and are developed and revised at a rapid rate, your best bet is to check fitness magazines for reviews. *SHAPE* and *FITNESS* magazines are two of the better sources of information—both subject exercise videotapes to intense scrutiny before rating them. Videotapes produced in conjunction with the major aerobics instructor certification organizations will tend to be of higher quality, with more stringent safety standards than most. Recommended certification organizations are the American College of Sports Medicine, IDEA/The International Association of Fitness Professionals, ACE/American Council on Exercise, and AFAA/Aerobic and Fitness Association of America. An aerobics instructor certified by any of these organizations can also assist you in selecting a home workout video. Above all, remember that movie and television stars are hardly the most credentialed fitness experts around.

Water Aerobics

An offshoot of land-based aerobics, **water aerobics** was developed for its many unique benefits. Aerobics performed in a swimming pool offers an additional exercise choice for people who are prone to musculoskeletal injuries. These individuals benefit from the buoyancy of the water, which reduces joint stresses associated with weight-bearing exercise. This makes water aerobics a natural choice for overfat exercisers or those with arthritis. Additionally, *because water offers 12 times the resistance of air, muscles must work that much harder to perform the same movements they would make on land.* Also, the coolness of an aquatic environment helps dissipate heat for individuals more prone to heat strain.

Anyone who enjoys water, dancing, and music can combine them into a fun cardiorespiratory workout. Even people who don't like to go underwater can enjoy water aerobics, because their heads stay above water throughout a workout. The same combinations and steps used during land-based aerobics can be performed in the water, although at a slower pace. The music used during a water aerobics session will be much slower as well (120 beats per minute versus 130 to 160 beats per minute for land aerobics). Participants keep exercise intensity at a level adequate for cardiorespiratory conditioning by using as many muscles as possible, by making broad movements across the pool, and by keeping trunk and limb movements underwater to add resistance from the water.

Additional equipment can be used to increase heart rates that fall below the 50- to 85-percent HR reserve level. These include wearing baggy shirts and shorts to increase drag and wearing webbed hand gloves or holding fans and buoys to pull and push against the water. "Aquacisers" wear special shoes for water sports that protect the soles of their feet from rough-textured pool bottoms. Even step aerobics (see the next section) has taken to the water with special underwater benches. And some water aerobics exercisers work out in the deep end of a pool, where standing is impossible, by wearing flotation vests or belts to keep themselves upright while they perform rhythmic movements and even jog in place or across the pool.

Water aerobics may offer psychological benefits to would-be exercisers not yet comfortable with their bodies. Because bodies are submerged throughout a workout, no one looks clumsy or out of place. Also, swim suits are not required. In fact, shorts and T-shirts not only provide extra drag, as mentioned previously, but also conceal modest people on their way to and from the locker room.

A word of caution when joining a water aerobics class: Make sure the instructor's goals are the same as yours. Many classes claim to feature "water aerobics" but do very little to condition the cardiorespiratory system. The majority of these classes spend time isolating specific muscle groups and performing exercises meant to increase muscular strength and endurance. There is nothing wrong with these exercises; in fact, they are a wonderful addition to a cardiorespiratory workout. However, the heart rates achieved with these exercises do not reach and/or maintain the 50- to 85-percent HR reserve level. Don't be afraid to ask an instructor to focus on continuous, rhythmic, large muscle movements if a class has been promoted as a cardiorespiratory endurance workout.

Step Aerobics

Since step aerobics was created in the 1980s, it has become as popular, if not more so, than its predecessor, aerobics. Men certainly have accepted step aerobics much more openly. Often called bench aerobics, **step aerobics** is regarded as a low-impact, high-intensity activity. Keeping one foot always in contact with either the bench or the floor, participants step on and off a bench 4 to 12 inches tall using a variety of leg and arm movement combinations. Movements facing the step mainly involve muscles from the front and back of the hip and thigh. Straddling the step involves the outer and inner thigh muscles to a much higher degree. Calf and shin muscle groups are recruited every time you step up and down. Upper body involvement can be as much or as little as needed to reach your target heart-rate range.

As with other aerobics programs, there are still questions about the risk of injury for people susceptible to knee and hip problems. Many physicians believe that step aerobics is too demanding for those starting out on an exercise program. This may be true, but if participants follow a proper progression, they seem to be at no more risk than for any other fitness activity. In fact, if bench height is correct, the muscle groups surrounding the knee and hip joints should become more conditioned as a result. Correct bench height creates a bend in the knee no deeper than a right angle when the foot is flat on the bench. Each base added to a bench to adjust height usually raises the bench 2 inches. Experiment with these bases to find the correct bench height for your stature and cardiorespiratory endurance level.

The foot's contact with the bench should be heel-ball-toe or flat-footed, while the return to the floor should be toe-ball-heel. Posture is maintained either upright or bent slightly forward at the hip joint, not the spine. Frequently changing the starting foot helps you avoid placing undue stress on one leg. And as with most forms of exercise, the shoe choice is critical. Aerobics shoes or special step aerobics shoes provide cushioning and shock absorption where it is needed most. Careful attention to these details will help minimize injury risk while maximizing the workout potential.

The tempo of the music used during step aerobics is around 120 to 124 beats per minute. This allows for movements in an optimal range of motion for the leg and hip joints. The rate of injuries may increase when movements become too fast and out-of-control. If an instructor is using music that feels too fast to you, request a music tempo to which you can complete a more intense, full range of movements to keep your heart rate in the target range.

Step aerobics is an excellent choice for home workouts. The cost of a bench is very low compared to other cardiorespiratory equipment—usually less than $120. Be sure to choose a quality bench, not one of the soft foam or "rebounding" models. The cushioning action may actually cause more knee joint injuries due to hyperextension, while the springlike benches may actually increase the impact on the return to the floor. Benches are portable and lightweight and can be stored under beds or in closets. They can be placed in front of a television for workouts to a variety of exercise tapes or while watching a favorite program. Step aerobics combined with more recent lateral training devices, or slides, offer an excellent cross-training workout. Try alternating step aerobics with the slide for equal periods of time (such as 2 minutes each) throughout a cardiorespiratory session. Virtually every lower-body muscle group should be involved to a high degree, and target heart rates may be more easily maintained.

Rope Skipping

Rope skipping is an excellent way to keep coordination and movement skills in tune. If you want to try jumping rope, choose a good rope long enough to reach from armpit to armpit while passing under both feet. The models with plastic disks that slide around the rope provide a good balance and weight to the rope.

If you are out of condition, do not try to do too much too soon (of course, this is good advice no matter what form of exercise you choose). Wear shoes with lots of cushioning for the ball of the foot because that is your landing point. Keep your arms relaxed near your sides, and let your wrists turn the rope. Beginners can skip (step-hop) with each revolution, while more advanced jumpers need to hop only once per revolution. Rope skipping does place

TABLE 6.3		
Rope Skipping (at 80 rope turns per min.)		
Step	Load	Total Jumping Time
1	Start with six 20-second bouts with a 10-second rest interval between each; in each succeeding workout, add 2 sets until you can do 12 sets; then go to the next step.	2 – 4 min.
2	Start with six 30-second bouts with a 10-second rest interval between each; in each succeeding workout, add 2 sets until you can do 12 sets; then go to the next step.	3 – 6 min.
3	Start with five 45-second bouts with a 15-second rest interval between each; in each succeeding workout, add 1 set until you can do 12 sets; then go to the next step.	4 – 9 min.
4	Start with six 1-minute bouts with a 30-second rest interval between each; in each succeeding workout, add 1 set until you can do 12 sets; then go on to the next step.	6 – 12 min.
5	Start with four 2-minute bouts with a 30-second rest interval between each; in each succeeding workout, add 1 set until you can do 8 sets; then go to the next step.	8 – 16 min.
6	Start with four 3-minute bouts with a 30-second rest interval between each; in each succeeding workout, add 1 set until you can do 8 sets; then go on to the next step.	12 – 24 min.
7	Start with four 4-minute bouts with a 30-second rest interval between each; in each succeeding workout, add 1 set until you can do 8 sets; then go on to the next step.	16 – 32 min.
8	Try to sustain skipping for 10 minutes; then rest for 2 or 3 minutes. In each succeeding workout, try to skip comfortably for as long as you can, up to 10 minutes. Eventually your goal is to complete three 10-minute bouts of skipping.	10 – 30 min.

concentrated and rigorous demands on the ankles, knees, and hip joints. However, keeping your jumping height within 1½ inch off the ground can minimize this stress. As you progress from beginner to more advanced, increase your workout intensity either by increasing the rope speed from 80 revolutions per minute to more than 120 or by using a weighted rope. A metronome or music with the right tempo can help you establish your speed.

We have observed that the heart rate of out-of-shape people comes close to maximum after only 1 to 2 minutes of continuous jumping. Quite often, they fatigue quickly and have to stop. Even people who are capable of running for 30 minutes have difficulty jumping for 10 minutes because of the constant demand on the relatively small calf muscles. You might consider incorporating jumping rope into a cross-training program involving shorter durations of a variety of activities in succession. Table 6.3 outlines a beginner's rope skipping program.

In-Line Skating

One of the fastest-growing sports in America with the potential to improve cardiorespiratory endurance is in-line skating. Many city and country streets are filled with people wearing these above-ankle boots sporting a straight row of four or five wheels. The popularity of in-line skating can be attributed in part to its playful nature and its speed. Skaters can enjoy the fresh air while exercising outdoors or take to the halls and concourses of indoor stadiums during poor weather. In-line skating is low-impact and involves the large muscle groups of the hips and thighs. The more proficient skaters lean their trunks forward, almost parallel to the ground, which requires very strong trunk muscles (as beginners trying to emulate this posture quickly learn).

Intensity of exercise with in-line skating can be modified by adjusting the speed and the amount of muscle used to propel oneself and to maintain balance. Hills, of course, require increased work on the way up and more control and skill on the way down. Even beginner skaters can increase their energy expenditure by making leg movements forceful and wide-ranging. Skaters who swing their arms purposefully in opposition or hold them in typical racing position, with one arm behind the back, can also improve their form and increase their speed. A typical recreational in-line skater achieves 14 to 15 miles per hour. It may be difficult to maintain target heart-rate ranges at speeds any slower than this. The best way to improve your form and make the most of an in-line skating workout is to take lessons from a trained instructor. The sporting goods store where you purchase your skates may be able to make recommendations.

Many people avoid in-line skating due to its reputation as a dangerous sport. *There are very few other fitness activities in which wearing safety equipment is so imperative.* Helmets and elbow, wrist, and knee pads are musts to prevent everything from scrapes to broken bones to brain damage. Do not underestimate their importance, and do not even think of purchasing in-line skates if you cannot also afford quality safety equipment. Additionally skating skill and technique lessons greatly reduce your chances of injury. Braking skill obviously should be one of the first things you master before hitting the streets. When you feel more comfortable and can remain relaxed while you are skating, you can more easily absorb bumps in the road. This confidence can go a long way toward keeping you on your feet—or should we say, wheels?

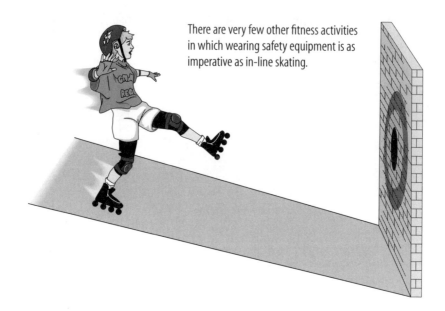

There are very few other fitness activities in which wearing safety equipment is as imperative as in-line skating.

In-line skating can be combined with other outdoor cardiorespiratory endurance activities for unique cross-training. Heading out for a 20-minute run that loops back to your skates, quickly changing equipment and then heading out for a 20-minute skate, and then looping back to your bike for a final 20-minute ride offers an excellent high-impact/low-impact/nonimpact combination workout.

Cardiorespiratory Endurance Exercise Equipment

According to the National Sporting Goods Association, Americans spend well over $1.8 billion on home exercise equipment each year. You can spend as little as $3 for a jump rope and as much as $3,000 for a computerized stationary bicycle system or even $8,000 for a motorized treadmill. Although commercial fitness centers, corporate fitness facilities, and university athletic centers offer the opportunity to work out regularly on stationary bikes, treadmills, rowing machines, stair-climbers, and other cardiorespiratory endurance machines, home versions of all types of equipment are becoming plentiful.

Purchasing exercise equipment for your home has become easy—and risky—thanks to the many infomercials aired on television. There are literally dozens of exercise devices from which to choose. Do your homework and consult with a fitness specialist prior to any purchase. Do not be one of those peo-

---

WAY OF LIFE
Cardiorespiratory Endurance Exercise

Don't be afraid to try a variety of activities when training for cardiorespiratory endurance. It makes your workouts fun, prevents overtraining, and keeps you motivated.

---

ple who hope that fancy equipment will make exercising easy. When this does not happen, the item ends up collecting dust in a corner. In fact, a large market has developed for barely-used second-hand fitness equipment, which tends to be available at relatively low prices. It is also important to exercise on quality equipment to benefit from your workouts. Suffice it to say, the $99 specials do not hold up well. With the better exercise machines today, you can easily and accurately adjust the work loads to meet your personal fitness needs.

The principles stressed throughout this book still apply when using cardiorespiratory endurance equipment. Make sure the exercise device allows you to work most of the large muscle groups continuously and rhythmically. The exercise must be rigorous enough to elevate the heart rate to your target range. Newcomers to exercise may need to experiment with a variety of equipment and activities to find the "perfect fit." Even the experienced walker, runner, swimmer, or cyclist needs the occasional alternative or diversion these machines offer.

One attraction of these machines is their ease of use. Most of the pieces are built to accommodate all levels of fitness ability. Each machine has a computer display area, some of which are quite extensive. For example, some machines have you enter your age and weight, choose a workout program, select the effort level, and in some cases choose an "opponent" whose machine is linked to yours for some friendly competition. Many machines have consoles that display number of calories expended, pace, distance covered (in miles or kilometers), and heart rate. If calories expended are displayed, be aware that unless you are asked to supply your own body weight for the calculation, the expenditure is based on a "typical user," such as a 150-pound male. Thus, if you are not asked to supply your body weight, consider the information simply a rough approximation. In general, pulse monitors that slip onto the earlobe or fingertip are not highly accurate. You would be advised to check their accuracy against your own manual pulse check before relying on them during your workouts. Such "bells and whistles" tend to entertain and motivate the user. But remember, no matter how sophisticated the machine, you still have to do the work.

The following is a brief overview of some of the more popular pieces of fitness equipment for developing and maintaining cardiorespiratory endurance.

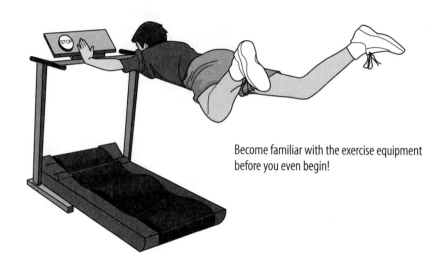

Become familiar with the exercise equipment before you even begin!

Treadmills

For some people, using a treadmill beats exercising outside in the dark or in bad weather. The treadmill features a belt that rotates as the person walks or runs on it. A treadmill typically utilizes a motor to move the belt, requiring the exerciser to maintain the selected pace. The price for a basic model of this type starts at around $1,000. However, less expensive, non-motorized models are also available, requiring the exerciser to move the belt during walking or running. The intensity of a workout can be readily controlled by adjusting the speed or the incline of the belt. Walkers and runners who want to train on hilly terrain can actually create their own hills by manipulating the height and increasing the duration exercised on the incline. Setting the treadmill at an incline is one way to elevate the heart rate into the target range. It also allows increased use of the "climbing muscles"—the quadriceps on the front of the thighs and the gluteals (buttocks). For additional motivation, a programmable treadmill varies the speed and incline automatically over a preselected period of time, working within specific intensities of your target heart-rate range.

When starting a treadmill, hold onto the frame and straddle the belt before pressing the power button. "Paw" at the belt with one foot to get an idea of the speed before stepping onto the belt with both feet. Prior to shutoff, most treadmill motors return the speed to a very slow pace. Not only does this allow you to gradually decrease your speed at the end of a workout, but it also ensures that the treadmill will not restart at too fast a pace for the next workout. Once you are on the treadmill and have your balance, release your hands from the rails and allow them to swing naturally by your side in opposition to your legs. Stay up toward the front of the treadmill and keep your focus forwards. In case you begin to stumble or lose pace, most treadmills are equipped with a large, bright red emergency/panic button. Locate this button before you even step on the treadmill so that you can quickly press it if the need arises. It beats flying off the end of the belt!

Because one foot is always in contact with the belt, walking on a treadmill is a low-impact activity, just as it is on land. Running on a treadmill or on land is a high-impact activity in that at some point, both feet are off the ground. Some treadmill manufacturers claim that their treadmill "gives" through slight flexing of the bed. However, it is questionable whether this feature reduces the impact forces enough for individuals experiencing overuse injuries to have a safe, comfortable workout. It may be more advisable to choose a nonimpact activity while recovering from impact-induced pains.

Stationary Bikes

The advantages of a stationary exercise bike are many. You can sip water, watch the news, or even read as you cycle. Also, if you are experiencing an overuse injury from a weight-bearing exercise such as walking, running, or dance aerobics, this nonimpact activity is a good way to maintain your cardiorespiratory endurance as you recover. For cross-training, consider alternating a day of running outside with a day of indoor cycling. Another idea is to combine the stationary bike with one or more machines in a single workout session to balance your fitness program.

A good exercise bike typically costs between $600 and $3,000. The less expensive models rely on resistance (how hard it is to pedal) from a flywheel with a belt on it or a fan wheel that generates air resistance. The resistance can be accurately adjusted, and these bikes are usually equipped with ergometers that measure the work performed. Some bikes are dual action: The handlebars can be pumped back and forth to exercise the arms, chest, and back while pedaling. Just make sure you actually pull and push instead of simply resting your hands on this type of handlebar. Electronic bikes allow you to choose both your resistance and a comfortable pedal frequency, with the work load generally measured in watts. However, the computerized displays make these bikes more costly.

For some exercisers, a recumbent bicycle may be a wise choice. Instead of sitting above the foot pedals, you sit in line with them, with your legs extended in front at the same level as your hips. This seating arrangement provides good back support and allows more involvement of the hip and thigh muscles.

A good exercise bike will weigh 50 pounds or more and will hold up well under heavy usage. You will definitely notice a smoother ride as you pedal the better-quality bikes. The seats are sturdy and easily adjustable. If the saddle that comes with the bike is not comfortable, you can purchase wider or narrower

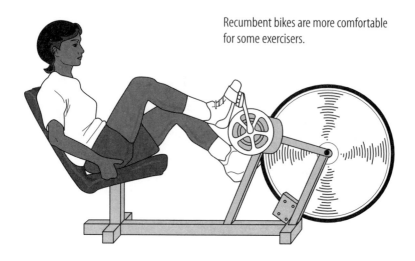

Recumbent bikes are more comfortable for some exercisers.

seats or padded covers that can be slipped over the current seat. As with a regular bicycle, make certain there is a slight bend in your knee when your foot has pushed the pedal down as far as it will go. If possible, use pedals equipped with foot straps so that you can maximize usage of the hip, thigh, and lower leg muscles.

Rowing Machines

Rowing is an excellent nonimpact activity for cardiorespiratory endurance. A good rowing workout involves the back, abdominal, arm, and shoulder muscles but places no high-impact stress on the hips, knees, and legs.

Rowing machines provide resistance in a similar manner to the stationary bicycles. The totally enclosed fan-wheel models, for which your intensity relies on how hard you row, are very popular. Good models closely simulate rowing as it is actually performed on water and cost around $700.

Machine rowing should simulate the actual work of rowing a boat. The push of your legs moves the seat back and forward on a metal frame while your arms pull a handlebar attached to a chain or pulley. Padded gloves offer protection against calluses. To begin the rowing movement, extend your legs gently at the hips and knees, and then complete a pull with your arms as your shoulder blades squeeze together. The recovery begins as you extend your arms toward the flywheel and then flex your knees and hips as the seat returns forward. The speed and the force with which you pull determines the resistance that you work against. It is important that your trunk remain mostly

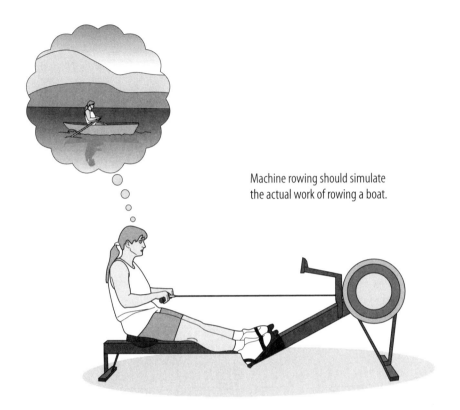

Machine rowing should simulate the actual work of rowing a boat.

erect throughout the movement. As with other cardiorespiratory machines, you can monitor your session in terms of time elapsed, calories used, work output, and distance traveled. Some models offer a cadence device to keep your actions smooth and rhythmical.

Stair-Climbing Machines

Who would ever have thought that climbing stairs would become a popular fitness activity? Today it's quite common to see a line of exercisers waiting to get on the stair-climbing machines at fitness centers around the country. Not only do stair-climbers offer a good cardiorespiratory workout, they rely on the leg and hip muscles to perform the work.

Some stair-climbers provide a nonimpact workout. Most popular is the "leg press" climber. This machine requires you to maintain contact with the pedals as one leg presses downward while the other leg and pedal recover. Another nonimpact climber is the recumbent machine, which provides some back

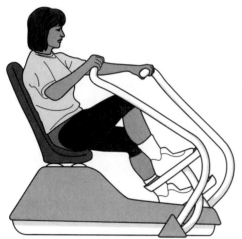

The recumbent stair-climber gives support to the back.

The leg press climber offers a nonimpact stair-climbing workout.

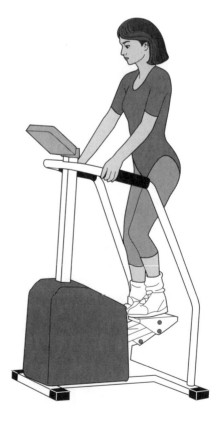

support. The feet maintain pedal contact while alternately pressing straight forward. Some models offer additional arm action involving the pushing and pulling of handlebars. A low-impact stair-climber is the "step mill," which acts much like an escalator, requiring you to alternately pick up your foot and transfer weight to a revolving step.

The stair-climber is most effective when you move your legs through their full range of motion, rather than using small, quick presses. Maintain an upright posture, and try to avoid leaning your body weight on the frame when you become fatigued. Newer models prevent you from making this form mistake by replacing typical handrails with an upright bar. Most machines can be programmed for various effort levels. For example, one model enables you to exercise at a rate of 4 to 17 times your resting energy level. You must keep your legs moving continuously on a stair-climber or the steps will "bottom out" (a subtle reminder for those who tend to occasionally slack off!). Although they are climbing to nowhere, this lack of destination doesn't seem to faze regular users. A good home model costs from $1,000 to $2,500.

Cross-Country Ski Machines

Can you guess which elite athletes have the highest maximal oxygen uptake values ever recorded? Cross-country skiers! Cross-country skiing offers the best potential cardiorespiratory activity because it involves every major muscle group and requires plenty of energy. During this nonimpact activity, the arm, shoulder, chest, and back muscles must pull and reach. The legs and hips must flex and extend in a wide range of motion. The trunk muscles must maintain erect posture and help the skier stay balanced. Indoor ski machines offer exercisers who lack access to snow a chance to master many outdoor skiing techniques while receiving an excellent cardiorespiratory workout. One exception is the technique of "skating." This is not possible on a cross-country ski machine due to the machine's parallel tracks, which retain the skis.

Skiing effectively does require some skill and balance. Some machines are equipped with a training rail to stabilize your upper body while you learn coordination, rhythm, and pace. You control the intensity of the workout through the speed of skiing, the resistance of the arm cords or poles, and the incline of the machine. Your arms alternately pull and recover in their fullest range of motion in front of and behind your trunk. Your legs fully flex forward and extend backwards, while your heels lift for that last big push. A good home model will cost from $500 to $1,200. One consideration for a home cross-country ski machine is whether the skis extend quite far beyond the rear of the machine or whether the skis are shortened. Keep this in mind when determining space availability for your skiing.

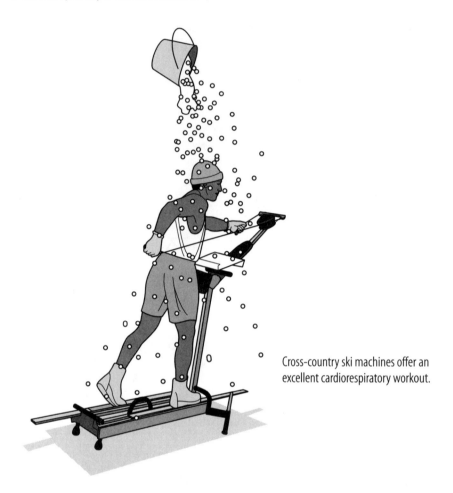

Cross-country ski machines offer an excellent cardiorespiratory workout.

Other Cardiorespiratory Endurance Machines

New exercise machines continually appear on the market, and a recent trend is to offer training devices that involve as many major muscle groups as possible. Devices like the SkyWalker, which suspend you while your legs and arms swing in a natural curve, are becoming popular as a nonimpact alternative. The difference between these machines and cross-country ski machines is a hydraulic system that offers resistance both on the push forward and the pull backward. This provides a benefit similar to that found in swimming, where the resistance of the water counters your every move.

Some exercise machines involve only arm movements. Arm ergometers use a rotary motion of the arms only, much the way riding a bicycle uses pri-

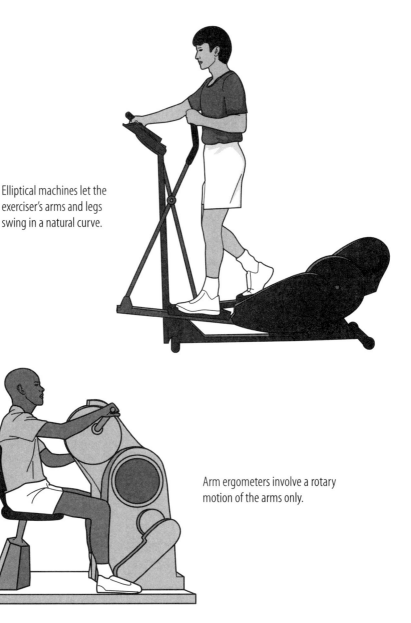

Elliptical machines let the exerciser's arms and legs swing in a natural curve.

Arm ergometers involve a rotary motion of the arms only.

marily the legs. Individuals who wish to develop cardiorespiratory endurance but who do not have full use of their legs find these machines very effective.

Cardiorespiratory endurance machines that require lateral movement of the legs, similar to skating, are gaining popularity. These "skating machines" involve the hip muscles in side-to-side movements instead of the forward-backward linear movements of walking, running, or biking. Skating machines

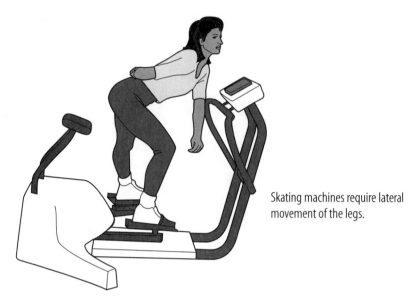

Skating machines require lateral movement of the legs.

can be combined with linear exercise machines for cross-training programs designed to lower the risk for overuse injuries. Interactive computer graphics programs accompany these machines and allow exercisers to "race" opponents through famous parks and boardwalks.

However, if you enjoy indoor skating but cannot afford the $1,000-plus price tag for a machine, $50 will buy you a slide board like those used in many group exercise classes. Slide boards range in length from 5 or 6 feet long for beginners to 8 feet or longer for more advanced sliders. The boards are coated with a surface that allows easy side-to-side gliding when wearing special booties over the shoes. Bumpers placed at each end of the slide board give a

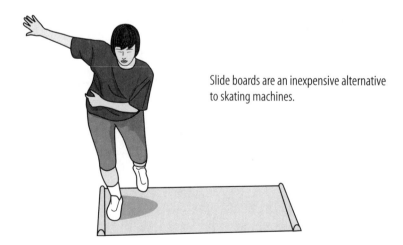

Slide boards are an inexpensive alternative to skating machines.

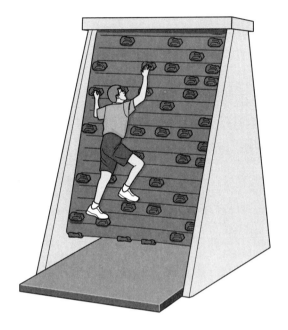

Treadwalls simulate actual rock climbing.

surface from which to propel oneself laterally. This activity can involve either low-impact or high-impact movements, depending on whether a jumping motion is used following propulsion off the bumpers. The board can be rolled up and tucked away in a closet when not in use.

Although rock climbing outdoors can be dangerous and is usually better left to the experts, it can be a great form of exercise. Many clubs are putting in indoor "climbing walls" equipped with safety ropes. For those squeamish about heights, there is even a "Treadwall," which mimics rock climbing without climbers getting more than 3 or 4 feet off the ground. Because the climbing holds are on a moving belt, climbers can "ascend" for as long as their arms and legs hold out.

WAY OF LIFE
Considerations When Choosing Cardiorespiratory Endurance Activities

- Comfort and fit of equipment
- Low-impact versus high-impact activity
- Water versus land activity
- Group versus individual activity
- Indoor versus outdoor activity
- Qualifications of exercise leader
- Cost of equipment or classes

With all the choices for cardiorespiratory endurance exercise available, it is practically impossible to come up with a valid excuse not to exercise these days. So find some activities and equipment that work for you, and get going!

Summary

You have a wide variety of activity choices to help you begin or expand your cardiorespiratory endurance program. Over your lifetime, you can base your choices on the form of exercise most suitable for your fitness level, your history of joint and muscle injury, and your personal tastes. As in walking and running, each of these activities must follow correct training specifics of intensity, duration, and frequency in order to elicit cardiorespiratory endurance benefits. And as always, any of the training specifics can be modified to suit your individual needs.

Key Words

AEROBICS: A variety of vigorous exercise routines and activities performed to music.

HIGH-IMPACT AEROBICS: Aerobics routines involving movements in which both feet may be off the floor at the same time.

LOW-IMPACT AEROBICS: Aerobics routines in which one foot is always in contact with the floor.

STEP AEROBICS: A low-impact, high-intensity form of aerobics that involves stepping on and off a bench ranging in height from 4 to 12 inches using a variety of step and arm combinations.

WATER AEROBICS: An offshoot of land-based aerobics; performed in a swimming pool.

A Way of Life Library

Burke, E. R. *High-Tech Cycling*. Champaign, IL: Human Kinetics, 1995.

Burke, E. R. *Science of Cycling*. Champaign, IL: Human Kinetics, 1986.

Carmichael, C., and E. R. Burke. *Fitness Cycling*. Champaign, IL: Human Kinetics, 1994.

Counsilman, J. E. *The Science of Swimming*. Englewood Cliffs, NJ: Prentice-Hall, Inc., 1968.

Gaines, M. P. *Fantastic Water Workouts*. Champaign, IL: Human Kinetics, 1993.

Kuntzleman, C. E. *Home Gym Fitness: Rowing Machine Workouts*. Chicago: Contemporary Books, 1985.

Powell, M., and J. Svensson. *In-Line Skating.* Champaign, IL: Human Kinetics, 1992.

Solis, K. *Ropics: The Next Jump Forward in Fitness.* Champaign, IL: Human Kinetics, 1992.

Thomas, D. G. *Swimming: Steps to Success.* Champaign, IL: Human Kinetics, 1989.

Town, G., and T. Kearney. *Swim, Bike, Run.* Champaign, IL: Human Kinetics, 1994.

CHAPTER 7

Developing Muscular Strength and Endurance

A muscle must be subjected to greater-than-normal loads to be strengthened. For most people, daily activities do not stimulate their muscles enough to cause strength and endurance increases. Even individuals who lead active lifestyles rarely participate in activities strenuous enough to elicit strength gains. Therefore, with advancing age, people typically lose strength. In fact, the loss of strength with age is so common that it traditionally was seen to be a direct result of the aging process. However, research now indicates that the majority of strength loss associated with aging is due to the lack of activities intense enough to maintain strength. Thus, as we grow older, we need to perform specific exercises of sufficient intensity on a regular basis to effectively develop and/or maintain muscular strength and endurance. These exercises are collectively known as resistance exercises. They force the muscles being worked to generate more tension by providing an additional resistance against which the muscles must act. The most common form of resistance exercise is weight lifting, but exercises using body weight (calisthenics) or elastic bands and partner-assisted exercises also provide resistance training.

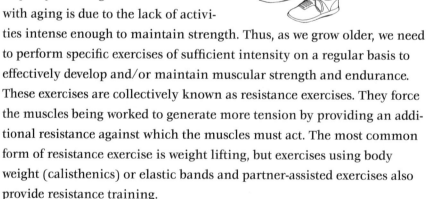

A s you read this chapter, keep these statements in mind:

- Strength improves when muscles are stressed systematically and progressively with a greater-than-normal load.
- Strength training increases muscle tissue and helps decrease body fat.

- Women who regularly weight train will experience increases in muscle mass, though not to the same extent as their male counterparts.
- Two to three training sessions a week generally can lead to significant strength gains.
- In many cases, the cause of lower-back pain is muscle weakness. A program of exercises directed at strengthening and stretching the muscles of the lower back and abdomen can do much to prevent or rehabilitate lower-back problems.
- Strength training programs that are not supplemented with cardiorespiratory training do not adequately develop and maintain good overall fitness.

Muscular strength, as mentioned in Chapter 1, is the ability of a muscle or group of muscles to generate maximal force. For example, the maximum amount of weight you can bench press one time represents the muscular strength of your chest, arms, and shoulders. Muscular endurance is the ability of a muscle or group of muscles to resist fatigue while either repeatedly generating forceful contractions or sustaining an isometric contraction. Muscular strength and endurance are discussed together in this chapter because resistance training can improve both. How, you may ask, does resistance training do this? Simply put, resistance training improves muscular strength, which in turn serves as the basis for muscular endurance. A stronger muscle is able to perform more repetitions with a fixed weight than a weaker muscle and therefore will demonstrate greater endurance. In this chapter, we discuss the training principles and guidelines for resistance training so you can develop an effective program for improving both muscular strength and muscular endurance.

Benefits of Muscular Strength and Endurance

Muscular strength is perhaps the most underappreciated and neglected component of physical fitness. Strong muscles often are seen merely as an attribute needed by athletes for maximizing performance. However, strong muscles not only improve athletic performance but also make work and leisure activities less taxing and more enjoyable. Thus adequate levels of strength have a positive impact on the quality of life. Although most people recognize the importance of cardiorespiratory exercise and its impact on health, few know about muscular strength and its role as a health-related component of physical fitness.

Strong muscles help prevent injuries in athletic competition and during daily activities by lending structural integrity to the joints they cross. The joints of the body are surrounded by muscles or the tendons of muscles, which help the ligaments hold the articulating bones together. The stronger the muscles, the greater their potential for resisting forces that could disrupt or injure the normal anatomy of the joint. In addition, strong muscles themselves are less prone to injury. The connective tissues that hold the muscles together, as well as attach them to the bones, become thicker, stronger, and less prone to tearing. The connective tissue harness becomes stronger because the connective tissue cells, like muscle cells, are stimulated by resistance training. They produce more collagen, which is the fibrous material that gives connective tissue its strength. The end result is stronger connective tissues that are more resistant to tearing or ripping whenever the muscles generate force.

Resistance training also leads to improvements in other components of physical fitness, such as local muscular endurance, muscular power, and body composition. As mentioned previously, muscular strength can improve absolute muscular endurance. For example, before strength training, you might be able to do 8 biceps curls with 70 pounds before fatiguing, but after six weeks of strength training, you might be able to perform 20 repetitions. In addition, strength training increases muscular power. Muscular power is also known as speed-strength because it depends on both speed of movement and the ability of muscle to generate force. Resistance training improves muscular strength and, as a result, can directly impact muscular power.

Resistance training also improves body composition by increasing lean body mass (muscle and bone) and decreasing fat weight. (To evaluate your body fat, see Chapter 3.) Some people who are not overly fat may actually gain body weight despite losing body fat with a resistance training program simply because muscle weighs more than fat. However, be careful! Large increases in body weight may mean you are consuming more calories than you are burning through exercise. Normally the increase in lean body mass due to strength training will not exceed 5 to 7 pounds over the course of a year's training.

An additional benefit of increasing lean body mass through resistance training is that it speeds up the body's metabolism. Exercise scientists know that the body must expend more energy (calories) to maintain muscle tissue than it does to maintain fat tissue. The increased metabolic rate not only results in loss of body fat but also makes it easier for individuals to maintain or control a favorable body composition.

Muscles also serve as the body's shock absorbers. They dampen the impact forces that normally occur during walking, running, and other activities. Without good shock absorbers (that is, strong muscles), over time these impact forces can damage the cartilage in joints. This may ultimately result in degenerative diseases such as osteoarthritis. In addition, strong muscles can help prevent common ailments such as lower-back pain. It is well documented that one of the key contributing factors to lower-back pain is poor muscular strength, specifically in the abdomen and lower back. Common remedies for back pain, such as heat application or medication, don't target the primary

- Increases muscular strength
- Increases local muscular endurance
- Increases muscle mass
- Increases bone density
- Increases connective tissue strength
- Prevents injury
- Helps maintain a favorable body composition
- Improves physical appearance
- Improves quality of life

cause—which for many individuals is weak muscles. But if muscular weakness is the problem, resistance training offers a long-term solution rather than a short-term treatment.

Finally, resistance training is also an effective way of building strong, dense bones. This is particularly important for individuals who have been diagnosed or are at risk for osteoporosis, a disease resulting in porous, brittle bones. All too often, we think of bone tissue as "lifeless" because that is how it is presented. In anatomy laboratories, the bony skeleton hangs in the corner, its bones white, dry, and lifeless looking. However, it is important to remember that in living, breathing individuals, the bones are made up of living cells, just like all the other tissues in the body. And as with muscle and connective tissue cells, bone cells respond to resistance training by making the bone tissue denser and thus better able to support loads and resist fractures.

In this chapter, we will present guidelines for developing muscular strength and endurance. Keep in mind that the focus is not on developing large, bulky muscles, as in body building, but on building stronger muscles. Combining strengthening exercises with your chosen cardiorespiratory endurance activities will further improve your physical fitness and help you get the most out of life.

Resistance Training Misconceptions

Although resistance training in various forms has been practiced for over 2,500 years, most of our current strength training practices are based on research performed since the 1960s. Despite the growing popularity of resistance training among men and women, however, there is still a lack of scientifically established training guidelines. Many training practices have stood the test of time in the sense that they must work or they would not still be around. Unfortunately many misconceptions have been perpetuated as well.

One misconception is that resistance training will make you muscle-bound, inflexible, and slow. All of these would be disastrous to any athlete or physically active individual. In truth, a properly designed and executed resistance training program will do just the opposite. Not only can it increase flexibility, it can improve muscular strength and endurance, speed, and jumping ability. In fact, many of the world's fastest athletes use strength training to enhance their performance. Not only that, Olympic weight lifters are second in flexibility only to gymnasts.

Keep in mind that *strength training and bodybuilding are not the same.* Strength training is not going to make you the next Arnold Schwarzenegger. Although individuals involved in both these activities perform resistance exercises, strength trainers and bodybuilders train to attain different goals. The goal of competitive **bodybuilding** is to put on as much muscle mass and to get as large as possible. In fact, one of the reasons the muscle-bound misconception prevails is because most people incorrectly associate strength training with the large bodybuilders. **Strength training** is designed to make your muscles stronger, not more massive. Bodybuilders spend many hours every day training to develop their muscles, whereas strength training may involve only 45 to 90 minutes of training two to three times per week. The amount of time most people spend in strength training simply isn't adequate for the increases in muscle mass produced by a bodybuilding workout.

Another common misconception is that women should not strength train because of its masculinizing effects. Certainly strength training can cause some **muscle hypertrophy,** or muscle enlargement, but it does not deepen women's voices or cause hair to grow on their chests. In other words, strength training does not cause increases in circulating levels of the male hormone testosterone. Remember, it is testosterone, not weight training, that controls masculinity.

Training Specifics

Mode: What Type of Exercise?

Muscular strength and endurance are increased through resistance exercises. Resistance exercises challenge the musculoskeletal system by increasing the amount of force necessary to perform a particular movement or activity. Weight lifting using **free weights**—barbells and dumbbells—is the most common form of resistance exercise. However, resistance exercises also can involve lifting other types of heavy objects, lifting body weight, pulling against elastic bands, and even pushing or pulling forcefully against immovable objects or training partners. Regardless of the type of resistance exercises used, as long as

---

WAY OF LIFE
Resistance Training Specifics

- *What type of exercise?* Resistance exercise using weights, elastic bands, machines, or body weight
- *How hard?* Use resistances allowing 10 to 15 RM
- *How long?* 45 to 90 minutes
- *How often?* Two to three times per week

---

the load is intense enough to stress the musculoskeletal system, the muscles will become stronger and the bones will become denser.

Resistance exercises involve two basic types of muscular contractions—static and dynamic. Static resistance exercises are called isometrics. In **isometric training**, no limb movement occurs during performance of the exercise despite the fact that the muscle is generating maximal force. An example of an arm and shoulder isometric exercise would be standing in a doorway and pressing your hands against the doorframe. Because no joint or limb movement is involved, isometric training is often used in clinical settings for rehabilitation after injury or surgery. Although strength gains resulting from isometric training have been documented, most authorities agree that resistance exercises involving movement (dynamic contractions) produce the best results. Thus the information presented in this chapter pertains exclusively to resistance exercises involving dynamic muscle contractions.

Dynamic exercises are resistance exercises that involve joint movement. The muscle actions causing the movement can be the result of either **concentric action** (muscle shortening) or **eccentric action** (muscle lengthening). The most common form of dynamic resistance exercise is known as **isotonic exercise.** It involves lifting a fixed amount of weight a specific number of times. Because most daily activities and sports involve dynamic types of muscle actions rather than isometric contractions, dynamic exercises are the most widely recommended.

Intensity: How Hard?

The difficulty or intensity of a strength training exercise is generally gauged by the load or resistance used during performance of that exercise. The intensity can be quantified as a percentage of your maximal strength, or as an x RM. RM stands for **repetitions maximum** and x denotes the number of repetitions performed. The term *repetitions* refers to the number of muscle contractions or lifts performed in succession without rest. For instance, if you lift a barbell weighing 100 pounds overhead 10 consecutive times, you have performed

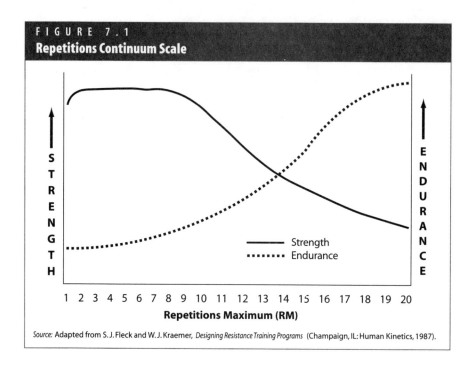

FIGURE 7.1
Repetitions Continuum Scale

Source: Adapted from S. J. Fleck and W. J. Kraemer, *Designing Resistance Training Programs* (Champaign, IL: Human Kinetics, 1987).

10 repetitions (reps). If after the tenth repetition the weight was so heavy that you could not perform or complete the eleventh repetition, then the 100 pounds would also be considered your 10 RM. Research has shown that the greatest gains in muscular strength occur when you train at your 2 RM to 10 RM weight load (which is roughly comparable to 75 to 95 percent of your maximal strength). If you are more interested in developing muscular endurance, then training at the 15 RM to 20 RM weight load would be appropriate. Obviously training in the 10 RM to 15 RM range will give you smaller, but still significant, gains in both strength and endurance (see Figure 7.1).

Duration: How Long?

Unlike cardiorespiratory training, strength training has no ideal length of time required for each session. The length of a training session depends on the number of muscle groups being trained, the number of **sets** and **repetitions** being performed, and the amount of rest taken between each set or exercise. A strength training program for the average person may take only 45 minutes, while for a trained athlete it may take 90 minutes. The time taken between sets and/or exercises, more than any other factor, affects the length of the workout. Unfortunately, again, there is no ideal rest interval between sets or exercises. The rest time between sets should be long enough for you to feel recovered before starting your next set—perhaps 2 to 3 minutes. The amount of rest taken when changing to another exercise can be shorter—perhaps 1 to 2 minutes—if you structure your program such that you train opposite muscle groups in sequence. For example, after finishing the bench press, you would perform seated rows, or after performing biceps curls, you would train the triceps. Obviously putting a little thought into the order in which you perform exercises can affect your training time.

Frequency: How Often?

You must get adequate rest between workouts to enable your body to recover before the next training session. Generally 48 hours between workouts is recommended, which means three training sessions per week. Research shows that this frequency of training can lead to significant increases in muscular strength, especially in untrained individuals. Note, however, the growing evidence that as little as two training sessions per week can be just as effective. This allows for increased recovery time between workouts and gives you more training time for improving other components of physical fitness.

Other Resistance Training Guidelines

In addition to these training specifics, keep in mind the following simple guidelines to make training even safer and more effective.

Breathing

When strength training, avoid holding your breath. Very often when lifting weights, people inhale deeply and then begin holding their breath, in what is known as the **Valsalva maneuver.** This maneuver causes dangerous fluctuations in blood pressure, with an initial rapid increase in blood pressure followed by a rapid decrease. In fact, if you continue to hold your breath for too long, you can suffer **weight lifter's blackout.** This occurs because the heart is not able to pump enough blood to the brain. Thus it is important to make a conscious effort to breathe while lifting. A rule of thumb is to "exhale with effort." That is, you want to exhale when lifting the weight or moving the weight stack upward against gravity and to inhale on the return phase when the weights or weight stack are being lowered.

Maintaining Proper Lifting Speed

There is no universally accepted speed of movement to use when strength training. As a general rule, the lifting phase of the repetitions should be faster than the lowering phase. One school of thought suggests that if it takes 2 seconds to lift the weight, it should take about 4 seconds to lower it back to the starting position. Regardless of the lifting speed you decide to use, it is critical

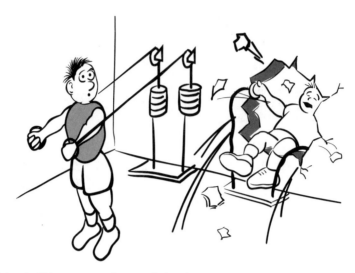

It is critical that the lifting movement be controlled at all times.

that the movement be controlled at all times. No bouncing or use of momentum during the performance of the exercise should occur. Bouncing movements do nothing to improve your strength, and more important, they can lead to serious injury.

When performed correctly, strength training can actually improve flexibility. The key is to use proper form and to move the resistance through the full range of motion. All too often, individuals can't move the resistance through the full range because it's too heavy or they don't know how to perform the exercise correctly. Using slightly less resistance and taking a little time to learn how to perform the exercise correctly will go a long way toward ensuring the success of your program. Seeking help from individuals certified by the National Strength and Conditioning Association (i.e. certified strength and conditioning specialist or certified personal trainer), the American Council on Exercise (i.e. certified personal trainer), or the American College of Sports Medicine (i.e. health fitness instructor or advanced personal trainer) is good advice.

Keeping Records

You should always keep accurate training records. Keeping track of training resistances, exercises, sets, repetitions, and machine settings is a great way to save time and to keep yourself motivated. Keeping records maintains your perspective by allowing you to look back and see how far you have come and how much you have gained. Seeing the payoff of your labor serves as an excellent motivator to maintain your lifelong fitness program.

Avoiding Injuries

The best way to avoid injuries when strength training is to maintain correct technique during each exercise. It is beyond the scope of this book to discuss specific techniques for all the resistance exercises that can be performed. As a result, we strongly recommend that you consult a certified fitness professional and/or refer to the resources in A Way of Life Library at the end of this chapter. Bouncing weights off your body or the weight stack, using momentum to help you perform a lift, and contorting your body into different configurations to lift a weight are all excellent ways to injure yourself. It's important to remember not to sacrifice form for weight.

Another safety tip is to train with a partner, particularly if you are lifting barbells and dumbbells. A training partner can serve as a **spotter** to help you complete a repetition, to lift weights off racks, or to hand them to you once you are ready to begin. A training partner can also be an excellent source of motivation.

Always perform an active warm-up of the exercise you are about to perform. An active warm-up involves performing a practice set of the specific exercise using a light weight (approximately 50 percent of your training weight). Doing so gives you a practice run in the exercise and helps warm up the specific muscles and joints about to be worked.

Balancing Your Workout

Finally make sure your strength training program is balanced. In other words, train opposing muscle groups equally. Avoid the temptation to exclusively train only certain muscles. The musculoskeletal system works by having muscle groups oppose one another. For example, the biceps muscle of the upper arm bends the elbow while the triceps muscle straightens the elbow. It is important to maintain a strength balance between opposing muscles because imbalances can lead to injury.

Clothing, Accessories, and Equipment

Clothing

If you have flipped through any fitness magazines lately, you are undoubtedly aware of the many ads pushing various types of training apparel and equipment. How much, if any, of this do you actually need for strength training? No special clothing is required for strength training because it is generally performed in the controlled environment of a health club, gym, or home. The most important factor is whether the clothing is comfortable and nonrestrictive.

The clothes can range from comfortable sweatpants and T-shirts to the more expensive Lycra warm-up outfits or Spandex shorts. Although the type of clothing worn is not of utmost importance, wearing it is. Strength training without shirts can be dangerous and unsanitary. The vinyl upholstery covering most weight benches and pads on machines becomes quite slick when wet, which can lead to injuries. Furthermore, it is extremely unpleasant to perform an exercise on a bench soaked with someone else's sweat. Be courteous. Wear clothing that is absorbent and/or carry a towel around with you to wipe down the pads and benches when you are done.

No special shoes are required for strength training. Just make sure to wear some kind of footgear to help protect your feet from injury and to prevent the spread of certain infections. The shoes should have a firm sole and give good lateral and arch support. Although running shoes are okay, tennis, basketball-type, or cross-training shoes are best.

Accessories

Some people consider wrist and knee wraps, wrist straps, gloves, chalk, and lifting belts to be standard equipment in strength training. Not so. Except for gloves, you don't need any of this equipment. In fact, we discourage its use.

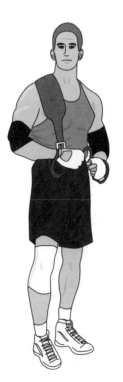

The general fitness enthusiast does not need wraps, straps, or belts to resistance train.

Wraps, straps, and belts are frequently used more as crutches to lift additional weight than they are for safety. Most fitness professionals recommend that a strength training program should involve loading the muscles within the limits of good exercise technique without dependence on joint wraps (knee and wrist). Doing so ensures that the muscles and the supportive connective tissues are challenged by the training and adapt in a balanced manner.

Likewise, except in instances when training with near maximal loads (that is, weights that can only be lifted one to five times), lifting belts are not recommended. Lifting belts assist the abdominal and oblique muscles in squeezing in on the abdomen to increase intra-abdominal pressure. This increased pressure helps to redistribute some of the load off of the vertebral column when lifting. However, if lifting belts are always used for support during training, the abdominal muscles will not be challenged to get stronger. Then in daily activities, for which a lifting belt is not worn, the weak abdominals may not be able to support the spine adequately. Obviously the consequences can be costly and painful. Remember, keep the use of lifting belts to an absolute minimum.

Free Weights and Resistance Training Machines

Free weights are the most common type of resistance training equipment. Free weights include barbells, dumbbells, bars, and weight plates. This equipment is relatively inexpensive and can be purchased at most sporting goods stores. Free weights are frequently sold in sets that include a steel bar that is 5 to 7 feet long, various weight plates ranging from 1.25 to 45 pounds each, and collars for holding the weight plates on the bar. A 300-pound set of weights typically sells for about $200. Dumbbells are the small weighted handles that you hold in each hand. They range in size from 1 to 100-plus pounds and are generally sold by the pound, with the cost ranging from 45¢ to 75¢ per pound. Consult with a fitness expert to determine which types and how much free weight equipment you need for resistance training at home.

Today most high school, university, corporate, and commercial fitness centers provide some type of resistance training machines. One advantage of such equipment is the ease with which you can change the weight loads (weight stacks are accessible from the exercise position) and adjust the equipment to suit your body size. Each piece of equipment usually has a placard mounted in a visible position with step-by-step instructions and illustrations. Most important, strength machines are safer than free weights and do not require a spotter. The smooth performance of the equipment and its ease of use allow for quick and efficient workouts.

Home versions of these exercise machines are also available at most sporting goods stores. If you are interested in purchasing one for your home, expect to spend anywhere from $1,000 to $3,000 for a good machine. You should try the machine out, making sure it adjusts to your body size and that it operates smoothly. It is always wise to get a fitness expert to help you pick out the best machine for your needs. Whether you have access to free weights or machines, the principles of training (see Chapter 4) are the same. A dynamic resistance training program should systematically, progressively, and regularly impose demands on your muscles to develop strength.

Muscle Adaptations to Resistance Training

The physiological changes that occur over the course of a training period (say, six to eight weeks) are referred to as training adaptations. If you repeatedly challenge and stimulate your muscles in the proper manner, you will see beneficial changes in your musculoskeletal system. Besides the obvious improvement in strength and endurance, the most outwardly observable adaptation to a strength training program is the enlargement of the trained muscles, or muscle hypertrophy. Muscle hypertrophy is believed to be primarily the result of enlargement of the thousands of cells that compose the muscles. Because the muscle cells are having to generate greater forces, they respond by producing more contractile proteins. These contractile proteins are directly responsible for the muscle cells' force-generating capabilities. By making more contractile proteins, each muscle cell becomes larger and stronger, which in turn makes the entire muscle larger and stronger.

There is evidence as well that the muscle cells not only become larger in response to resistance training but also increase in number. This is called **muscle fiber hyperplasia.** This increase in the number of muscle cells makes the muscle bigger and stronger. These findings conflict with the long-held belief that a person is born with a set number of muscle cells and that this number does not change throughout life. It should be noted that the extent to which muscle cell hyperplasia contributes to muscle hypertrophy in humans is unclear. Thus it is currently believed that individual muscle cell enlargement, rather than muscle cell hyperplasia, is the primary way in which the muscle gets larger and stronger.

The Effects of Resistance Training in Women

Some women fear that exercising with barbells and weight machines will make them overly muscular and unfeminine-looking. There is no scientific basis to this fear. The inherent capacity for muscle development is genetically determined by sex hormone levels. The male hormone, testosterone, causes muscle bulkiness in males. Even though this hormone is present in women, the amount is too low to have a substantial effect on muscle size. More and more women are now enjoying the improvements in body composition and shape that strength training affords them. In fact, nowadays it is not uncommon to see more women than men in the previously male-dominated weight room.

Although resistance training can cause some muscle enlargement in women, it has been erroneously touted by some equipment manufacturers as a means to increase breast size. Resistance training can increase the size of the chest muscles, but it does nothing for the breasts themselves. Heredity, body fatness, and pregnancy are the factors that determine breast size.

Exercises for Building Strength and Endurance

This section examines primary exercises for the muscles of the various regions of the body. Because a variety of resistance exercises can be used to work a particular muscle, examples of some of the more common ones are shown. If you do not have access to free weights or machines, we have also included partner-assisted exercises, calisthenic-type exercises, and exercises using elastic bands. Remember, if you are working with free weights a spotter should be present. Also, for all the exercises, it is imperative that you learn correct form and technique to avoid injury. If you are unsure about your form or technique, consult a fitness professional.

To put together a resistance training program, pick one exercise for each of the body regions and perform them in the order listed. If you are just starting, perform a light warm-up set of the exercise followed by a 1-minute rest, and one training set of 10RM. After two to four weeks, you can add a second training set, and after about eight weeks, you can add a third. For most people, three training sets is adequate to continue building muscular strength and endurance. A final note: Don't be afraid to periodically change resistance exercises. It adds variety to your workouts and ensures continued strength improvement.

1. Exercises for the Hips and Front of the Thighs

TECHNIQUE TIPS:

1. When performing squats and lunges, keep your lower back extended so that the normal curvature is maintained (do not round your lower back) throughout the exercise.

2. When performing squats and leg presses, place your feet shoulder width apart, with your toes turned out slightly.

3. Do not move your knees forward past your toes.

4. Do not exceed a 90-degree bend in the knees.

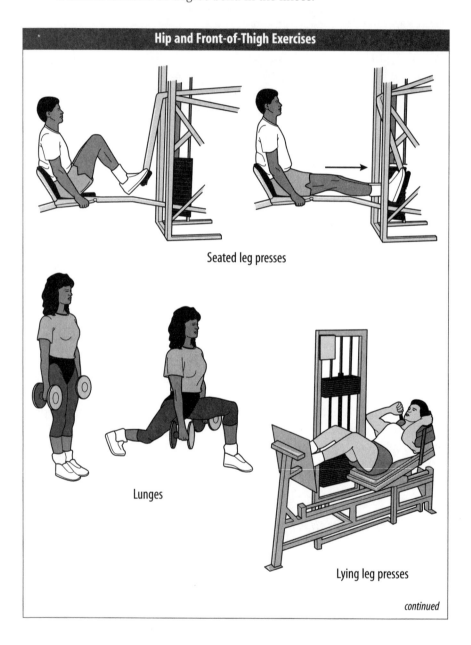

Hip and Front-of-Thigh Exercises

Seated leg presses

Lunges

Lying leg presses

continued

Hip and Front-of-Thigh Exercises *(continued)*

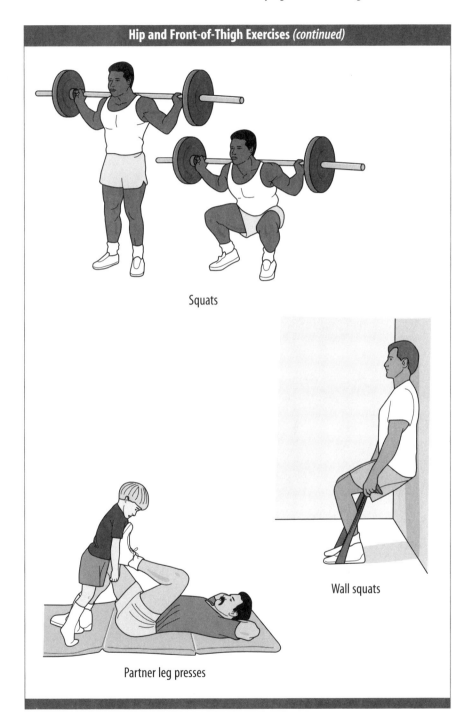

Squats

Wall squats

Partner leg presses

⛷ *2. Exercises for the Back of the Thighs*

TECHNIQUE TIPS:

1. When performing the prone hamstring curl exercises:
   - Do not allow your lower back to arch.
   - Do not hyperextend your neck by looking up. Rest your head on the bench, or keep looking down.

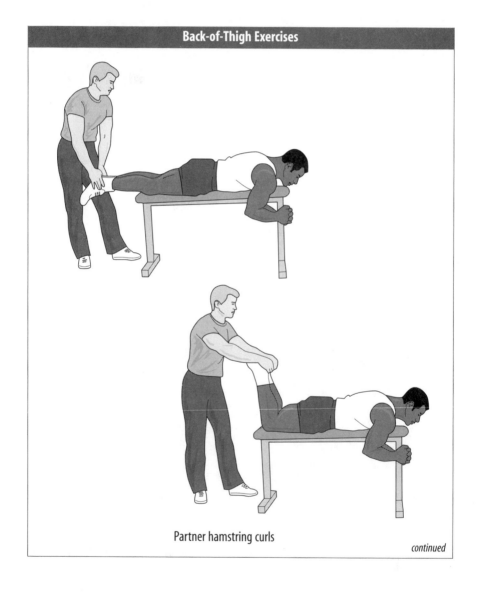

Back-of-Thigh Exercises

Partner hamstring curls

continued

Back-of-Thigh Exercises *(continued)*

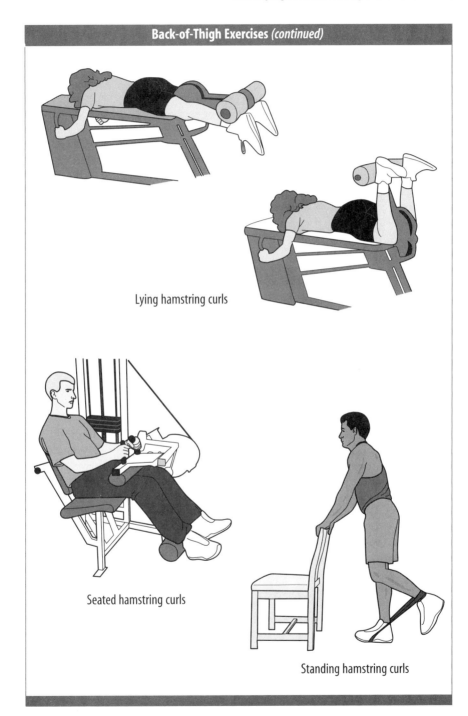

Lying hamstring curls

Seated hamstring curls

Standing hamstring curls

⚇ 3. Exercises for the Chest

TECHNIQUE TIPS:

1. Position your hands about shoulder width apart
2. When using a chest press machine, adjust the machine so that the handles are at about nipple level.
3. When using a barbell, do not bounce the bar off your chest.
4. Do not arch your lower back to complete the lift.

Chest Exercises

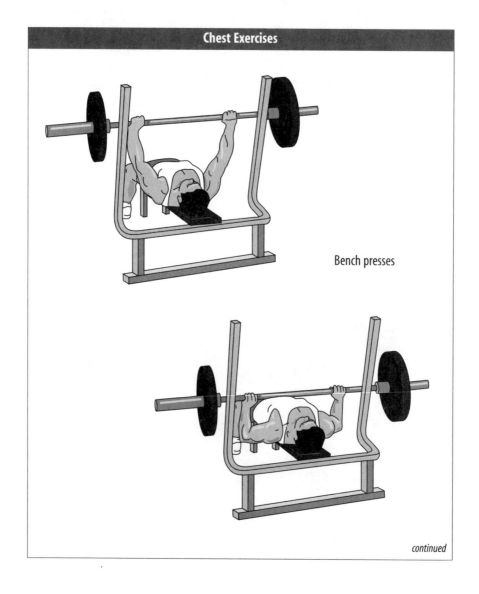

Bench presses

continued

Chest Exercises *(continued)*

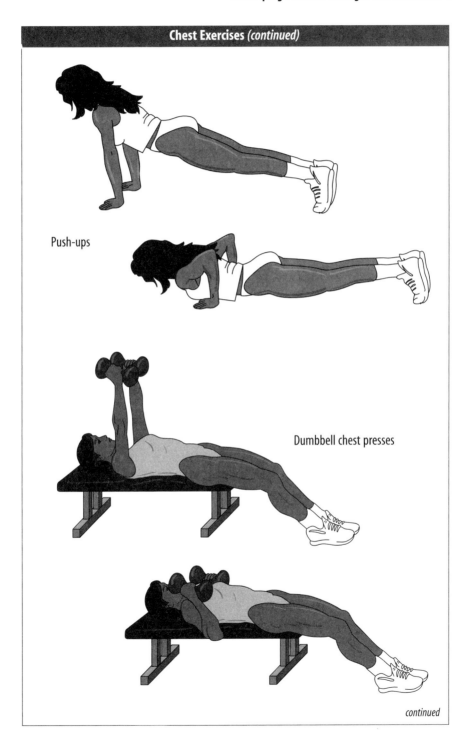

Push-ups

Dumbbell chest presses

continued

Chest Exercises *(continued)*

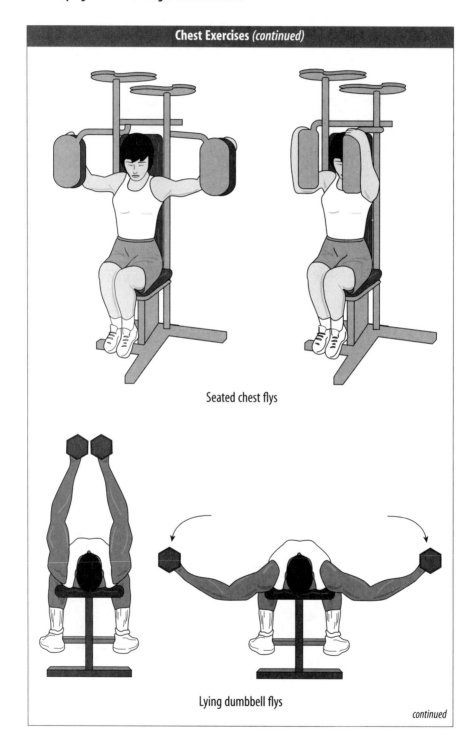

Seated chest flys

Lying dumbbell flys

continued

Chest Exercises *(continued)*

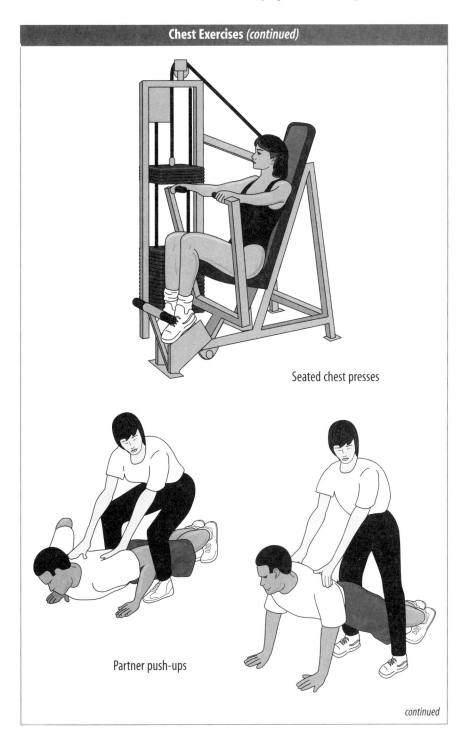

Seated chest presses

Partner push-ups

continued

Chest Exercises *(continued)*

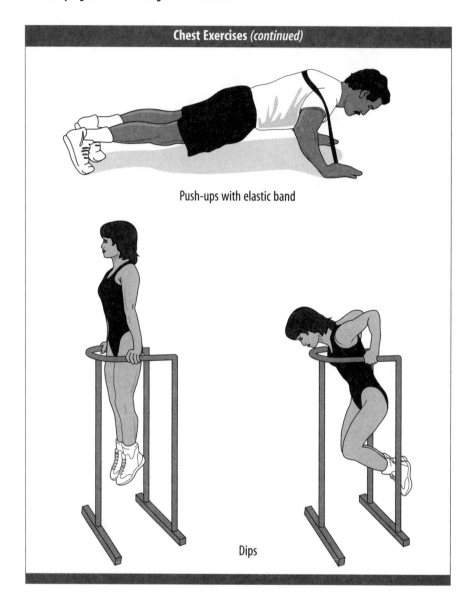

Push-ups with elastic band

Dips

⠇⅄ *4. Exercises for the Upper Back*

TECHNIQUE TIPS:

1. Concentrate on squeezing your shoulder blades together at the top position.
2. Do not arch your lower back to complete the lift.

Upper-Back Exercises

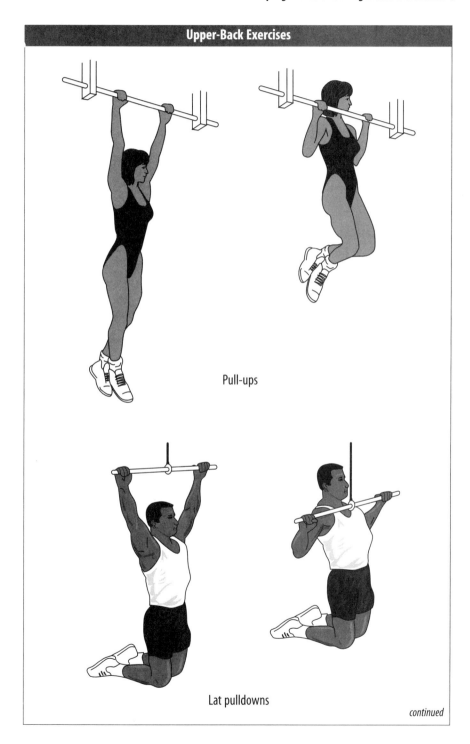

Pull-ups

Lat pulldowns

continued

Upper-Back Exercises *(continued)*

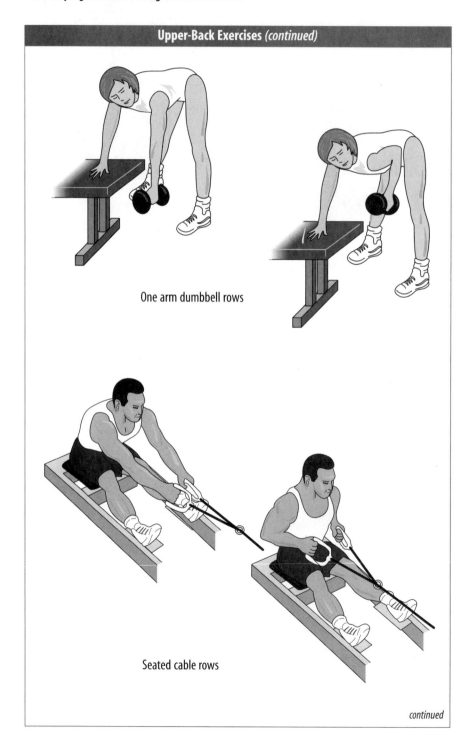

One arm dumbbell rows

Seated cable rows

continued

Upper-Back Exercises *(continued)*

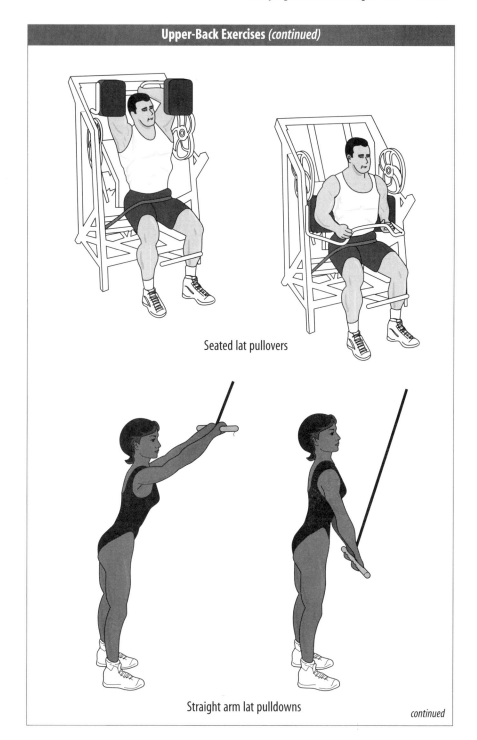

Seated lat pullovers

Straight arm lat pulldowns

continued

Upper-Back Exercises *(continued)*

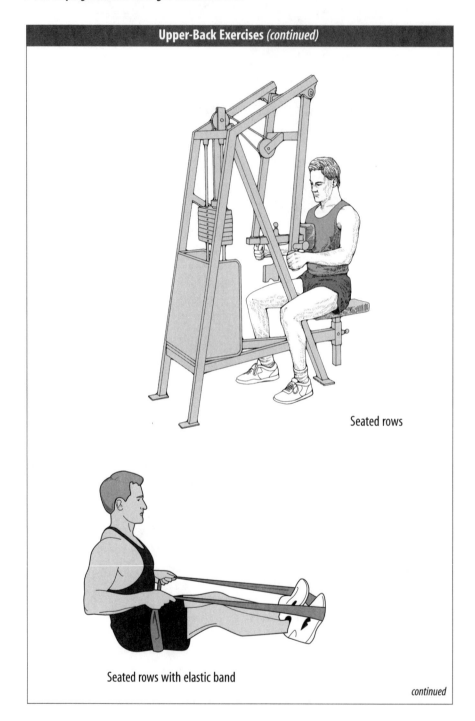

Seated rows

Seated rows with elastic band

continued

Upper-Back Exercises *(continued)*

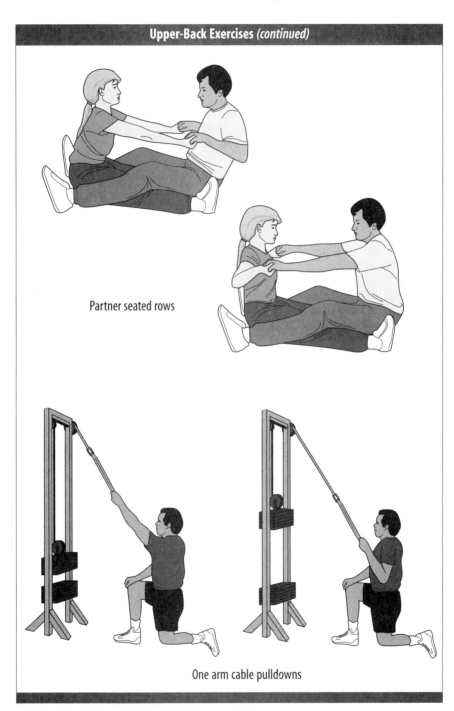

Partner seated rows

One arm cable pulldowns

☹⋏ 5. Exercises for the Shoulders

TECHNIQUE TIP:

1. When performing shoulder presses, do not arch your lower back to complete the lift.

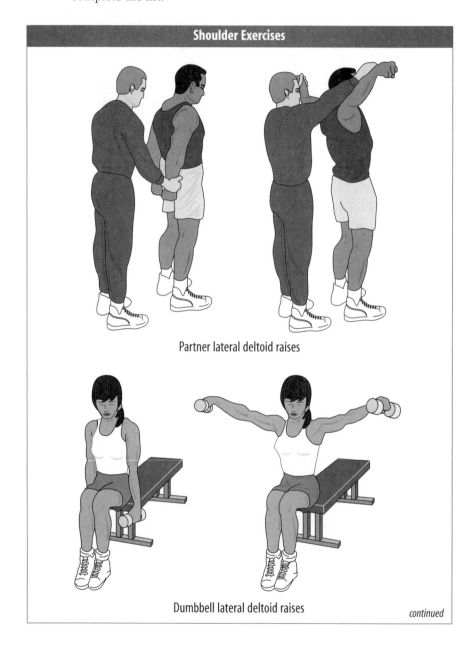

Shoulder Exercises

Partner lateral deltoid raises

Dumbbell lateral deltoid raises

continued

Shoulder Exercises *(continued)*

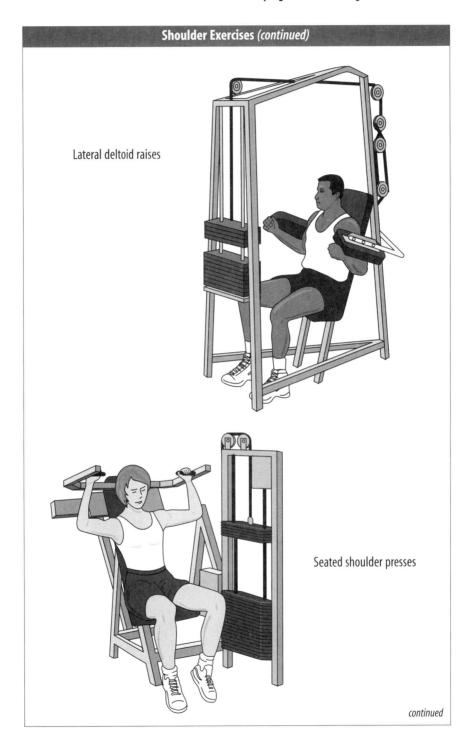

Lateral deltoid raises

Seated shoulder presses

continued

Shoulder Exercises *(continued)*

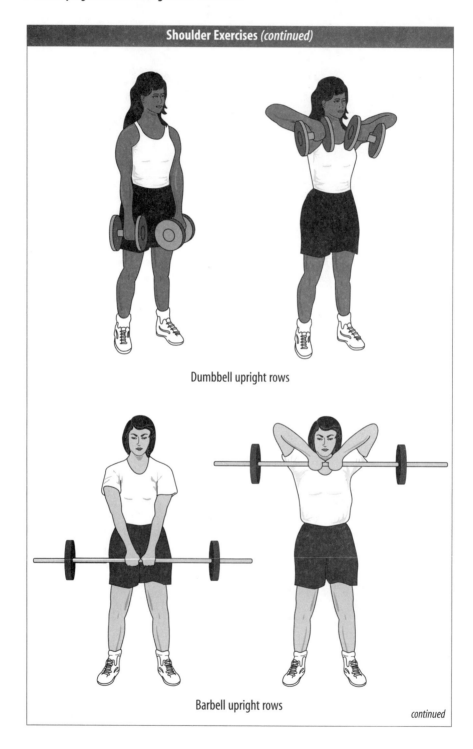

Dumbbell upright rows

Barbell upright rows

continued

Shoulder Exercises *(continued)*

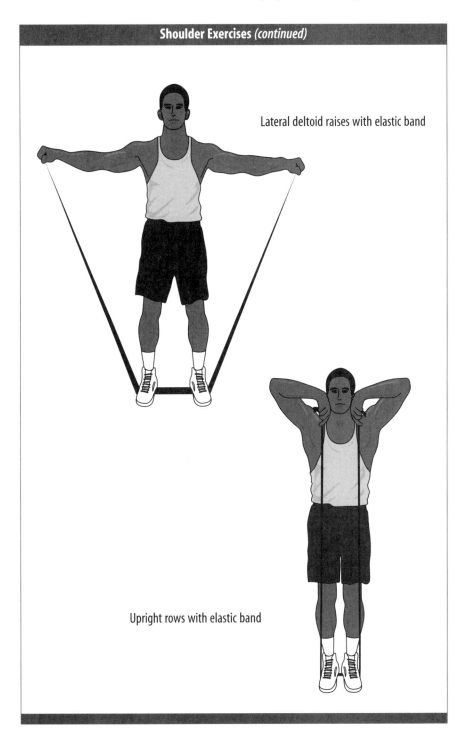

Lateral deltoid raises with elastic band

Upright rows with elastic band

6. Exercises for the Lower Back

Lower-back pain is a common complaint of many men and women. In general, the causes of backaches include poor posture, improper body mechanics, inactivity, excess body fat, and weak lower-back muscles. In many cases, appropriate exercises can eliminate the cause of back pain. According to statistics, about 80 percent of back pain is due to muscular weakness or inelasticity. Ruptured vertebral disks account for less than 5 percent of all cases of back pain.

TECHNIQUE TIPS:

1. When performing back extensions:
   • Do not arch (hyperextend) your lower back.
   • Do not hyperextend your neck.

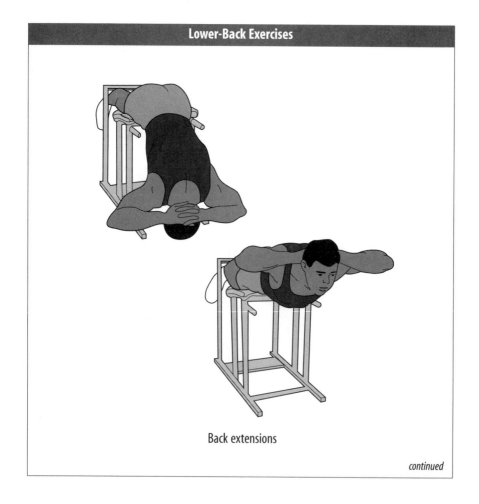

Lower-Back Exercises

Back extensions

continued

Lower-Back Exercises *(continued)*

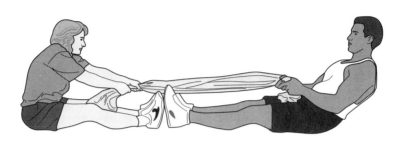

Partner back extensions

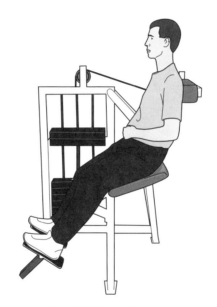

Seated back extensions

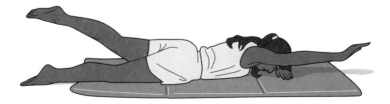

Lying alternating limb lifts

⁞⅄ 7. Exercises for the Abdominal Region

Whether you use weights or not, exercises for developing abdominal strength and endurance are a must in every physical fitness program. The abdominal muscles play a prominent role in maintaining correct posture and thus preventing lower-back pain. They also help stabilize the torso when performing work with the arms or legs. By stabilizing the torso, strong abdominals enable the muscles of the upper and lower extremities to generate more force. More force generated at the extremities can mean running faster, jumping higher, and changing directions quicker. It is no wonder that many coaches call the abdominal region the body's center of power.

TECHNIQUE TIPS:

1. Avoid pulling on the back of your head with your arms when performing crunches.
2. Do not do abdominal work with straight legs.
3. Do not arch your lower back off the mat at the end of each crunch. Concentrate on keeping your lower back pressed against the floor or mat.

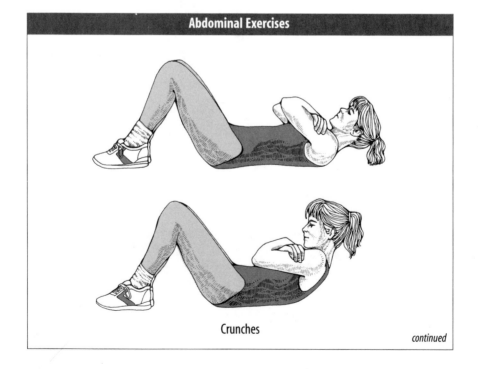

Abdominal Exercises

Crunches

continued

Abdominal Exercises *(continued)*

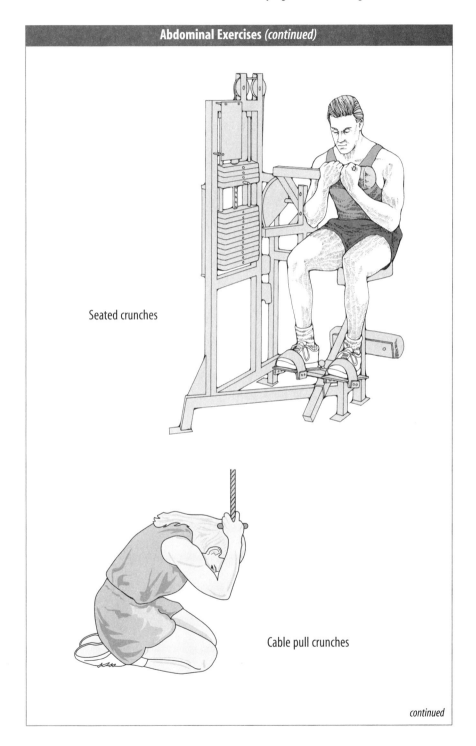

Seated crunches

Cable pull crunches

continued

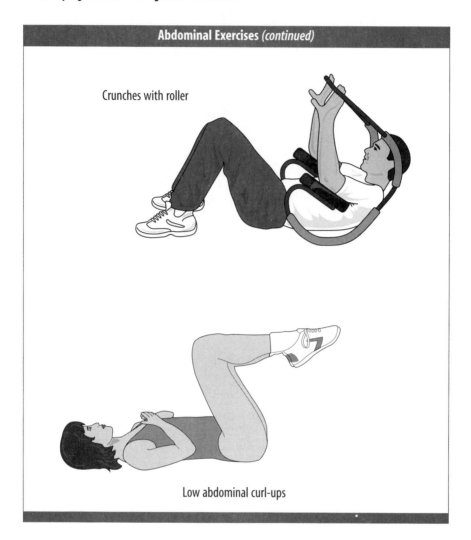

Abdominal Exercises *(continued)*

Crunches with roller

Low abdominal curl-ups

8. Exercises for the Side of the Trunk

TECHNIQUE TIP:

1. Avoid ballistic, twisting types of movements.

Side-of-Trunk Exercises

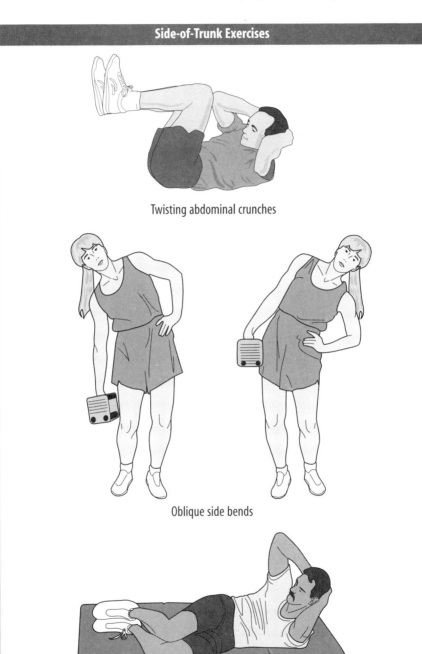

Twisting abdominal crunches

Oblique side bends

Side lying oblique crunches

continued

Side-of-Trunk Exercises *(continued)*

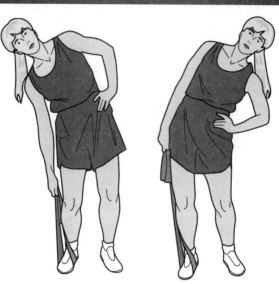

Oblique side bends with elastic band

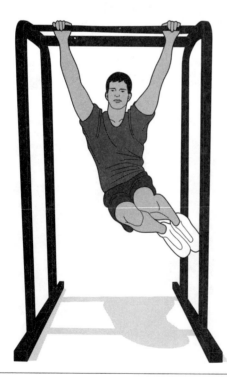

Hanging oblique crunches

continued

Side-of-Trunk Exercises *(continued)*

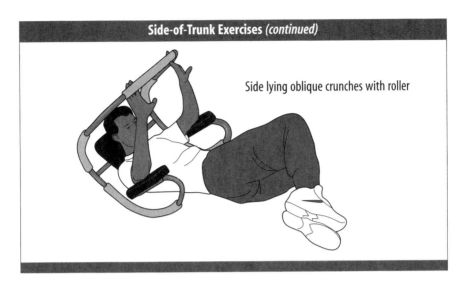

Side lying oblique crunches with roller

9. Exercises for the Front of the Upper Arms

TECHNIQUE TIP:

1. When performing arm curls, avoid arching your lower back to complete the lift.

Front-of-Upper-Arms Exercises

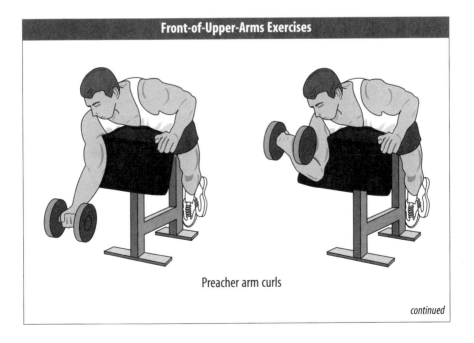

Preacher arm curls

continued

Front-of-Upper-Arms Exercises *(continued)*

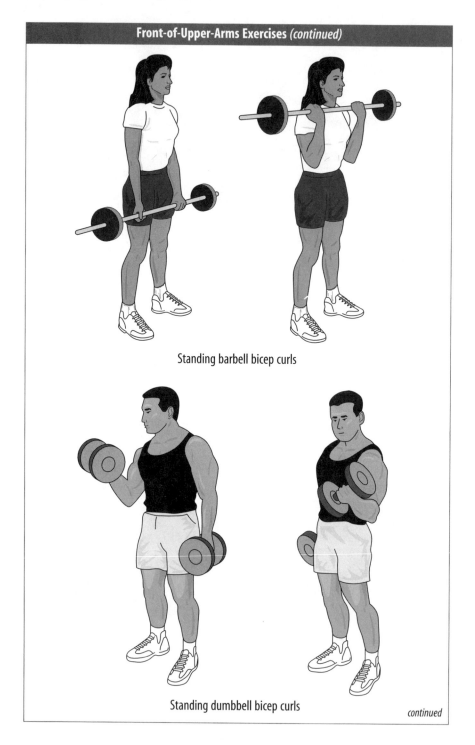

Standing barbell bicep curls

Standing dumbbell bicep curls

continued

Front-of-Upper-Arms Exercises *(continued)*

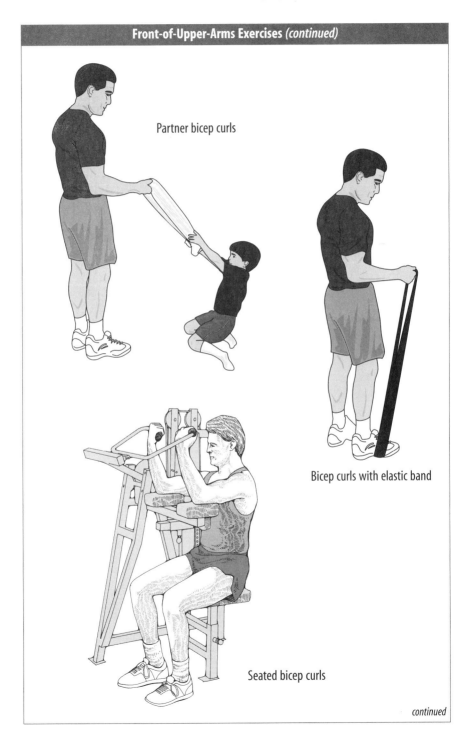

Partner bicep curls

Bicep curls with elastic band

Seated bicep curls

continued

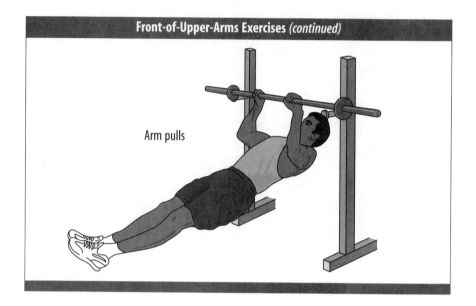

Front-of-Upper-Arms Exercises *(continued)*

Arm pulls

10. Exercises for the Back of the Upper Arms

TECHNIQUE TIPS:

1. When performing triceps press-downs, keep your abdominal muscles tight to prevent arching of the lower back.
2. When performing lying triceps extensions, keep your elbows pointing straight up towards the ceiling. Do not let them flare out.

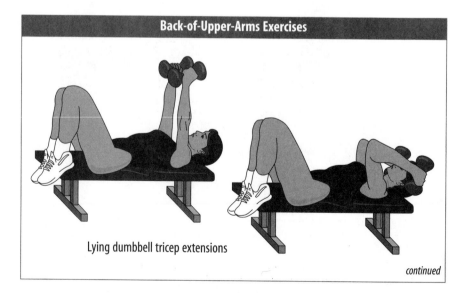

Back-of-Upper-Arms Exercises

Lying dumbbell tricep extensions

continued

Back-of-Upper-Arms Exercises *(continued)*

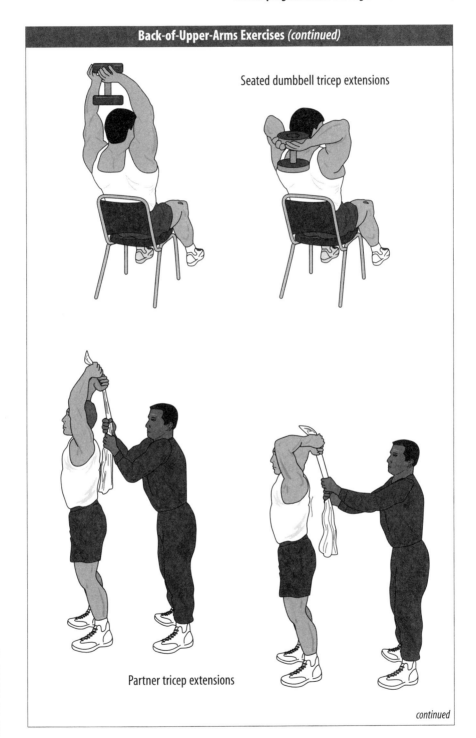

Seated dumbbell tricep extensions

Partner tricep extensions

continued

Back-of-Upper-Arms Exercises *(continued)*

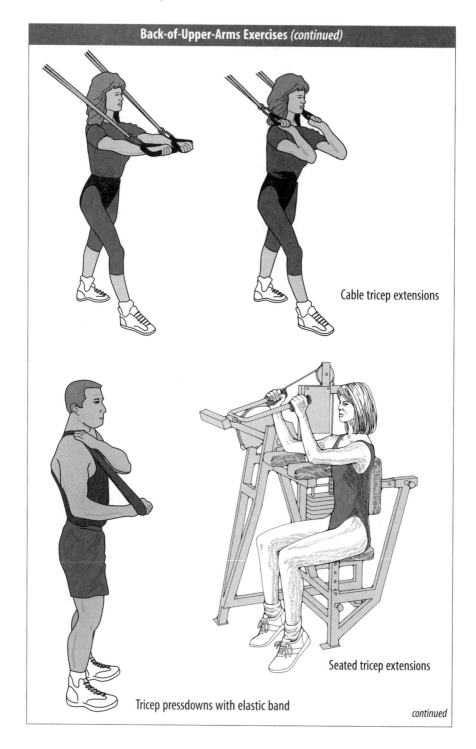

Cable tricep extensions

Tricep pressdowns with elastic band

Seated tricep extensions

continued

Back-of-Upper-Arms Exercises *(continued)*

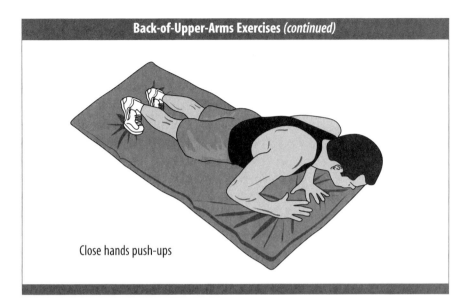

Close hands push-ups

:X 11. *Exercises for the Front of the Lower Leg*

TECHNIQUE TIPS:

1. Keep the exercise movement isolated at your ankles by not twisting your body or changing the position of your hips.

2. Avoid rapid, bouncing-type movements to prevent the straps or elastic bands from slipping off the top of your foot.

Front-of-Lower-Leg Exercises

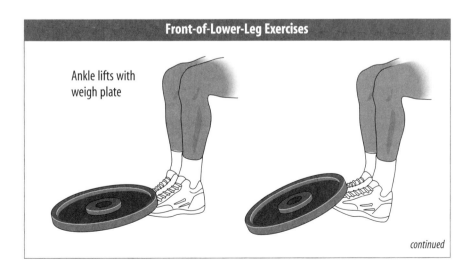

Ankle lifts with weigh plate

continued

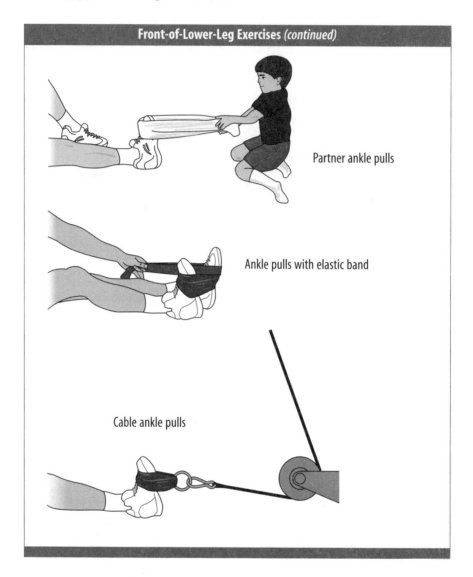

Front-of-Lower-Leg Exercises *(continued)*

Partner ankle pulls

Ankle pulls with elastic band

Cable ankle pulls

12. Exercises for the Back of the Lower Leg

TECHNIQUE TIPS:

1. When performing standing calf raises, do not lock your knees. Keep a slight bend in your knees to prevent overstressing the knee joint.
2. Avoid bouncing-type movements by keeping the up and down phases of the exercise slow and controlled.

Back-of-Lower-Leg Exercises

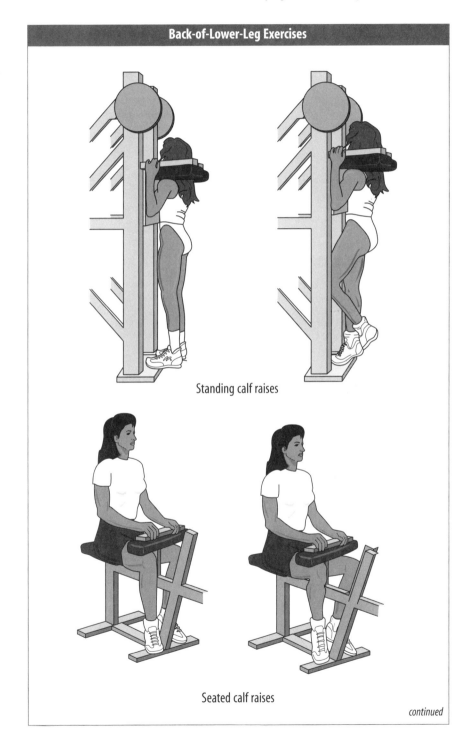

Standing calf raises

Seated calf raises

continued

Back-of-Lower-Leg Exercises *(continued)*

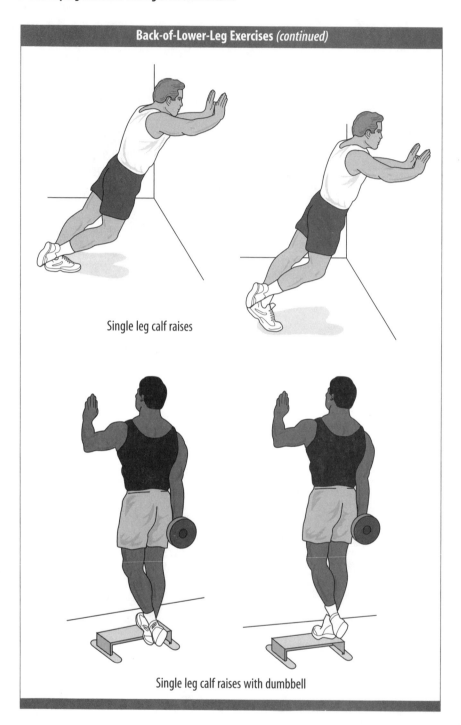

Single leg calf raises

Single leg calf raises with dumbbell

Summary

The benefits of resistance training are impressive. Research indicates that bones are both stronger and healthier when subjected to sufficient intensity of resistance training. Improved body composition (increased lean body mass) has always been recognized as a major benefit of strength training programs. The development and maintenance of muscular strength and endurance helps you to be more efficient throughout your daily living. Your posture is improved, and lifting, carrying, and moving heavy objects is easier. People with strong abdominal and back muscles tend to experience less lower-back discomfort. A regular program of strength building activities is highly motivating when it results in a firm, lean appearance. Also, people who possess good muscular strength, as well as balance and flexibility, tend to be less prone to injury during physical activity. Even walking, climbing stairs, or simply sitting can be less traumatic to the body if you have well-trained muscles. All things considered, possessing a good level of muscular strength and endurance is a necessity if you want to lead a robust, active life.

When you combine strength training exercises with the exercises for cardiorespiratory endurance (see Chapters 5 and 6) and flexibility (see Chapter 8), you have the ingredients for developing a personalized program that will not only get you in shape but help maintain excellent fitness and health. Remember that a safe, reasonable, effective program will help you feel better, look better, and function better.

Key Words

BODYBUILDING: A type of exercise progr designed specifically to cause as much muscle enlargement as possible. Bo uilding is also a sport in which the competitors are judged on muscle d opment and symmetry.

CONCENTRIC ACTION: A type of muscle actio which force is generated while the muscle shortens. Concentric muscle act are performed during the up-phase of a lift.

DYNAMIC EXERCISES: Exercises that involve joint ement.

ECCENTRIC ACTION: A type of muscle action in whi rce is generated while the muscle lengthens. Eccentric muscle actions ar rformed during the lowering phase of a lift.

FREE WEIGHTS: Equipment such as bars, plate weights, d bells, and barbells used in resistance training.

ISOMETRIC TRAINING: A mode of resistance training in whi e muscles generate force, but with no resulting joint movement.

ISOTONIC EXERCISE: A dynamic mode of resistance training in which the muscles generate force against a constant resistance, such as when performing a bench press with an 80-pound barbell.

MUSCLE FIBER HYPERPLASIA: An increase in the number of cells found within a muscle.

MUSCLE HYPERTROPHY: The enlargement of muscle, usually resulting from resistance training.

REPETITION: A single muscle contraction or lift.

REPETITIONS MAXIMUM (RM): The maximum load that can be lifted a given number of times. For example, 6RM refers to the maximum weight that can be lifted six but not seven times.

SET: A group of repetitions or lifts performed in succession without rest.

SPOTTER: A person who assists with safety, checks form, and encourages the lifter performing a resistance exercise.

STRENGTH TRAINING: An exercise program that is designed specifically to increase muscular strength.

VALSALVA MANEUVER: The act of holding one's breath, often when lifting weights. The Valsalva maneuver causes dangerous fluctuations in blood pressure and should be avoided.

WEIGHT LIFTER'S BLACKOUT: Passing out during weight lifting due to performing the Valsalva maneuver (breath holding).

A Way of Life Library

Baechle, T. R. *Essentials of Strength Training and Conditioning.* Champaign, IL: Human Kinetics, 1994.

Fleck, S. J., and W. J. Kraemer. *Designing Resistance Training Programs,* 2d ed. Champaign, IL: Human Kinetics, 1997.

Pearl, B., and G. T. Moran. *Getting Stronger: Weight Training for Men and Women.* Bolinas, CA: Shelter, 1997.

Peterson, J. A., C. X. Bryant, and S. L. Peterson. *Strength Training for Women.* Champaign, IL: Human Kinetics, 1995.

Westcott, W. L. *Strength Fitness: Physiological Principles and Training Techniques.* Madison, WI: Wm. C. Brown, 1995.

CHAPTER 8

Stretching for Flexibility

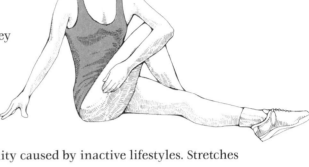

Millions of people lose the ability to bend, reach, and stretch as they age because their bodies are underexercised. Flexibility exercises (stretches) are designed to prevent or to remedy the inflexibility caused by inactive lifestyles. Stretches should be performed through a full range of motion on a regular basis. In this chapter, we will present a sequence of stretches that develop and maintain flexibility in all the major muscle groups.

As discussed in Chapter 4, fitness workouts should begin with a warm-up and end with a cool-down consisting of continuous low-intensity activity. It is important to gradually increase body temperature, heart and breathing rates, and blood flow to the working muscles before shifting into the more vigorous conditioning part of your workout. One of the best ways to warm up is to perform your conditioning activity at a low intensity (for example, slow walking and jogging before running). After 3 to 5 minutes of such movements, either perform stretches for all the major muscle groups or focus on specific muscles that feel particularly tight. If you feel loose enough to move your trunk and limbs through their full range of motion for your conditioning segment, you can stretch at other points in the workout. Stopping to stretch after you have warmed up for a cardiorespiratory endurance workout will necessitate an additional **mini warm-up** to return your heart rate to your target range before beginning the vigorous conditioning segment. You can concentrate more on stretching during your cool-down when you do not have to be concerned with keeping your heart rate in any particular range. Also, during the cool-down, your muscles and connective tissues are warm and pliable. Optimal stretching may be easier during your cool-down when you are more relaxed, not keyed up and ready to move. However, if you are performing muscular strength and endurance exercises, stretching between sets makes the most of your rest periods. You can still rest while you stretch, and this method saves you time by eliminating the need to stretch at the end of the workout. Your between-sets stretches may also improve the range of motion for the particular strength/endurance exercise being performed.

As you read this chapter, keep these statements in mind:

- Flexibility is an important, yet often neglected, physical fitness component.
- Stretching regularly may enhance your entire conditioning program by allowing your movements to be at their fullest possible range of motion.
- Stretches performed after a gradual, rhythmical warm-up help prepare your body for more vigorous activity.
- Stretches performed during your cool-down may be most beneficial due to the warmth and pliability of your muscles and connective tissues at this time.
- Bouncy, ballistic movements during stretching tend to cause reflexes that actually oppose the desired lengthening of muscles and connective tissues. Instead of bouncing or jerking, "statically" stretch slowly to a position of slight discomfort, and hold.

Benefits of Stretching

When you engage in fitness activities such as those for cardiorespiratory endurance, your trunk and limbs certainly move through a greater range of motion than if you simply sit around all day. However, even these moderate ranges of motion stop short of maximizing your **flexibility**—your ability to move your joints through their full range of motion. Stretching exercises, performed correctly, are safe and effective for developing your flexibility. Stretching promotes more comfortable movement through a full range of motion during all of your fitness activities, making them more fruitful.

Additionally, stretching all the major muscle groups helps reduce flexibility imbalances caused by using muscle groups on one side of the trunk or limbs more than the others. Frequently these flexibility imbalances, along with strength imbalances, lead to injury. A common example is the combination of tight lower-back muscles and weak abdominal muscles. The result of this imbalance frequently is lower-back pain. One useful approach to reducing lower-back pain combines stretches for the lower-back and hip flexor muscles, strengthening exercises for the lower-back and abdominal muscles, and posture education. Although stretching may not be the definitive answer to injury prevention, we do know that ensuring the fullest safe range of motion for all joints enables the body to move more freely during exercise and play.

Stretching exercises also can be used during relaxation sessions. As you overcome muscle and connective tissue tightness with stretching, your body becomes more at ease and comfortable. Combined with deep breathing, stretching just plain feels good!

Training Specifics

Mode: What Type of Exercise?

Increasing the range of motion of all the major joints in your body requires you to perform stretches that specifically target the muscles and connective tissues crossing those joints. If your goal is to improve your overall flexibility for well-balanced fitness, incorporate all 15 stretches described in this chapter. If you want to focus on a smaller number of body parts to begin with, that is fine. But to avoid flexibility imbalances and possible injuries in the future, introduce stretches for the opposing muscle groups as soon as possible.

Static stretching has been proven very effective for general flexibility. This means you move slowly to the stretch position and hold when you reach the point of slight discomfort. Notice that the word *pain* is not used here! For improvements in general flexibility, avoid bouncy, ballistic movements. **Ballistic stretching** may impose sudden strains on the muscles and connective tissues involved and trigger reflexes that actually oppose the desired stretching.

Intensity: How Hard?

Overstretching, especially if done with rapid movements, can lead to injuries. However, to improve flexibility using the overload principle, you have to ask your body to move to a point slightly beyond what is normally comfortable.

Therefore, during static stretching, move your trunk or limbs to a position that lengthens the muscles and connective tissues being stretched as much as possible. *Never stretch to the point of pain, but only to the point of slight discomfort.* Focus on relaxing as you hold the stretch. If you exhale as you move into the stretch position and then continue breathing normally as you hold, these exercises should be enjoyable and relaxing.

Duration: How Long?

Once you reach the point of slight discomfort with a static stretch, hold this position for at least 15 seconds. Many muscles and connective tissues benefit greatly from holding the stretch even longer, especially if the joints are unusually inflexible. Although it is perfectly acceptable to hold a stretch as long as you want, to get anything out of the stretch it must constantly be held at the point of slight discomfort. As you hold a stretch, you may find that your trunk or limbs loosen up considerably. When this happens, continue stretching at ever-increasing distances to maintain that slight discomfort.

Frequency: How Often?

Unlike exercises for the other physical fitness components, there is no limit to how often you can perform stretching exercises. If stretching is performed correctly, you do not run the risk of overuse injuries or not recovering from a previous stretching session. We recommend that you stretch at least three times per week for general flexibility and daily for the greatest improvements. These stretching exercises can be used before and after a conditioning workout, between sets of muscular strengthening exercises, or alone as a comprehensive flexibility workout. We also recommend that you stretch whenever you get a chance or whenever you feel your body tightening up. Once you become familiar with your muscles and their particular stretches, you can easily do them as you stand or sit, any time during the day. Such impromptu stretching may help you avoid tight muscles and may even refresh you.

Stretches to Avoid

Even the best flexibility program can be injurious if the stretches are performed incorrectly. Additionally careful reevaluation of certain traditional stretches that have been performed for years show them to provide a high risk for injury. The following represent some examples of exercises to avoid. As you will see, most of the problems with these stretches relate to the potential for overstretching and bending joints in ways for which they are not designed. For each contraindicated stretch, we have suggested less risky alternatives.

Yoga Plough

The original purpose of this exercise was to stretch the muscles of the upper and lower back and hips. Many researchers believe that this exercise can injure the nerves and vertebral discs in the neck and back region by using body weight to forcibly stretch the muscles. A safe alternative is the lower-back and hip stretch (exercise 8).

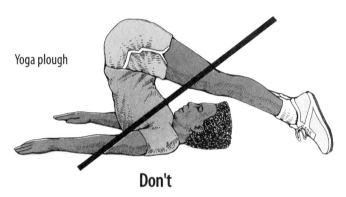

Yoga plough

Don't

Hurdler Stretch

This exercise has been used for years, especially by track athletes. It still may be appropriate for the highly trained hurdler or sprinter, but recent findings suggest that it puts abnormal stress on the inner side of the knee of the rear bent leg. These knee ligaments do not have to be subjected to such a stretch. Safe alternatives are the standing or lying quadriceps stretch (exercise 12).

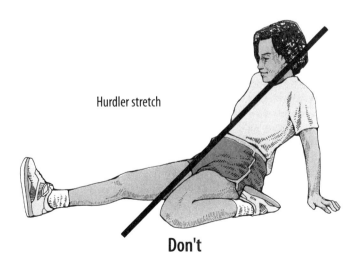

Hurdler stretch

Don't

Deep Knee Bends

It was common years ago to see football players waddling around performing deep knee bends or stretches in the full squat position. Many knee injuries have been attributed to this forcible bending of the knee joint with full body weight. The standing or lying quadriceps stretch (exercise 12) is recommended as an alternative.

Toe Touching

For years, toe touching or "windmills" were standard recommended daily exercises. Bending at the waist from a standing position and using upper-body weight and bouncing to touch the toes puts extensive stress on the ligaments and vertebral discs of the back. The hamstring stretch (exercise 13) is a safe alternative.

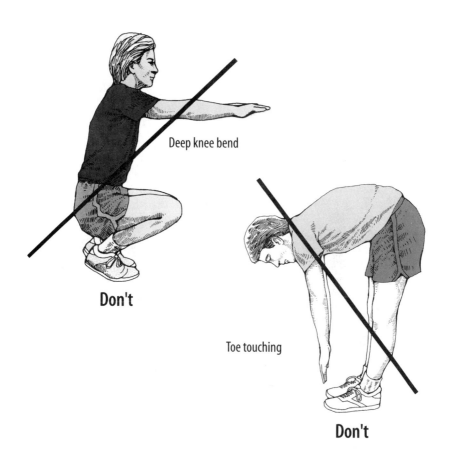

Deep knee bend

Don't

Toe touching

Don't

Neck Hyperextension or Full Neck Circles

When you drop your head back, either alone or as part of a circling motion, you risk damaging the nerves and vertebral discs of the neck. This is especially true of fast, uncontrolled neck circles. Safer alternatives are the rear and side neck stretches (exercise 1).

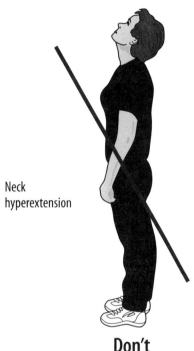

Neck
hyperextension

Don't

Clothing and Equipment

A major plus for stretching is that it requires no special clothing or equipment. It goes without saying that loose-fitting or stretchy clothing will allow you to move most comfortably in your full range of motion. When you perform exercises in the lying position, you might benefit from an exercise mat if a carpet or rug is not available. While stretching outdoors, use a tree for balance and the grass as a soft mat.

Individuals with near-optimal flexibility and for whom money is no object can enhance their range of motion with commercial stretching aids. For example, plastic devices that look like rockers fit under your feet to help stretch your calf muscles and Achilles tendons. A rope-and-pulley system that fits over a door stretches the hamstrings, quadriceps, and upper-body muscles. You may choose to use household items such as towels or ropes to enhance the range of

WAY OF LIFE
Stretching Basics

- Warm up with rhythmical, low-intensity movement before stretching.

- Stretch at the end of your workout during your cool-down, when your muscles and connective tissues are warmest and most pliable.

- Follow the suggested sequence of exercises; this will help you remember all the exercises.

- Do each exercise slowly and smoothly without bouncing.

- To improve your flexibility, hold stretches at the point of slight discomfort, not at the point of pain.

- Hold stretches for 15 seconds or more.

- Stretch at least three days per week, and stretch more often for optimal results.

motion of your stretches. Perhaps the cheapest stretching aid is a partner who takes your trunk or limb to the point of slight discomfort and either holds it or gives resistance. This does require clear communication between partners and a knowledge of safe support positions.

Flexibility Exercises

This section outlines stretches for all the major muscle groups. You can perform them in any order you desire. You may remember the flow better and not omit any stretches if you begin with your neck and progress down your body. Stretches can be performed either standing, sitting, or kneeling unless stated otherwise. For standing upper-body exercises, your knees should be slightly bent, and your feet should be shoulder width apart, with your upper body aligned with your pelvis. Remember, stretching should be smooth and controlled. Hold each stretch for a minimum of 15 seconds, and perform the stretch as many times as you feel necessary.

1. Rear and Side Neck Stretches

PROCEDURE:

1. Press both shoulders down, and maintain this depressed position throughout the stretch.

2. Lower your chin toward the middle of your chest, and hold for 15 seconds.

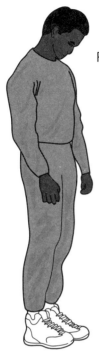

Rear neck stretch

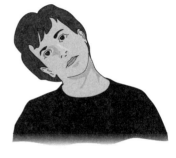

Side neck stretch

3. Move your chin approximately 2 inches to the right, continuing to aim it downward. Hold for 15 seconds before repeating the stretch approximately 2 more inches to the right. Hold for 15 seconds, and then continue in a path toward your right shoulder, holding every 2 inches for 15 seconds.

4. When you reach your right shoulder, hold for 15 seconds.

5. Rotate your head to a face-front position, and lower your right ear toward your right shoulder. Hold for 15 seconds.

6. Lift your head and repeat steps 1–5 moving toward your left shoulder.

2. Middle-Shoulder Stretch

PROCEDURE:

1. Stand with your right arm extended straight out to your side, thumb up and palm forward. Maintain this thumb-up position throughout the stretch.

2. Bring your right arm across your body in front of your chest. With your left hand just above your right elbow, gently pull your right arm farther across your body, and hold for 15 seconds.

3. Do not rotate your trunk. If needed for comfort, rotate your head left to look at your right hand.

4. Repeat with your left arm.

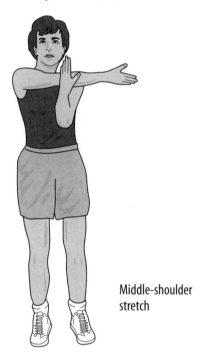

Middle-shoulder
stretch

3. Upper-Back and Rear-Shoulder Stretch

PROCEDURE:

1. Extend your arms in front of your chest, and cross one over the other so that your palms face each other. Interlock your fingers.

2. Lower your chin toward your chest.

3. Reach your arms forward as far as possible, moving your shoulder blades away from each other, and hold for 15 seconds.

4. Chest and Front-Shoulder Stretch

PROCEDURE:

1. Reach behind your trunk with both hands, and interlock your fingers. Keep your palms facing each other and your elbows slightly bent throughout the stretch. For some people, this is as far as a safe stretch should go.

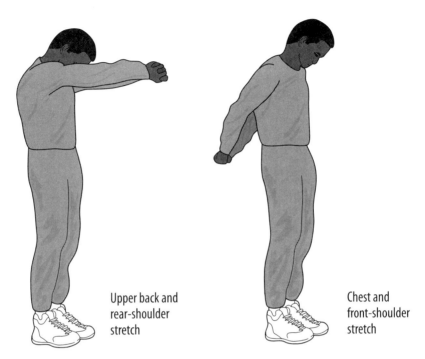

Upper back and rear-shoulder stretch

Chest and front-shoulder stretch

2. Lift your arms upwards, aiming for a position horizontal to the ground. Hold for 15 seconds.

3. Do not lean forward.

5. Triceps Stretch

PROCEDURE:

1. Lower your chin to your chest.

2. Lift your right arm straight up, and bend your elbow.

3. Place the palm of your right hand on your back between your shoulder blades.

4. Use your left hand to gently pull your right elbow toward the left. Hold for 15 seconds.

5. Repeat with your left arm.

6. Side Stretch

PROCEDURE:

1. Stand with your feet at least shoulder width apart and your knees slightly bent.

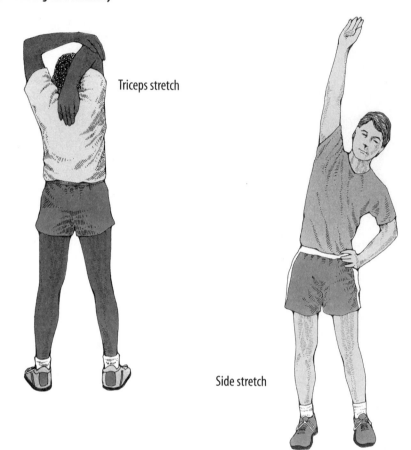

Triceps stretch

Side stretch

2. Place your left hand on your left thigh or hip for support.

3. Lift your right arm up in line with your right ear, and lean as far to your left as possible. Hold for 15 seconds.

4. Return your trunk to the upright position, and repeat to the right, beginning with your left arm lifted up.

7. Abdomen Stretch

PROCEDURE:

1. Lie face down on the floor, with your hands placed just outside your shoulders.

2. Look at the floor and maintain that head position throughout the stretch (not only is it safer for your neck, it also allows you to see how high your trunk has lifted).

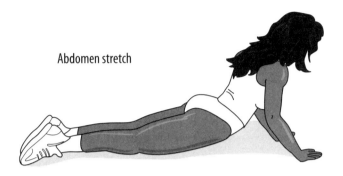

Abdomen stretch

3. Begin to straighten your elbows, arching your back slightly. (Note: If arching your back is painful, either lower your trunk to a more comfortable position or eliminate this stretch.)

4. Stretch only to the point where your navel begins to leave the floor, and hold for 15 seconds. Your pelvis should maintain contact with the floor throughout the stretch.

8. Lower-Back and Hip Stretch

PROCEDURE:

1. Lie on your back with your legs slightly bent at the knees.

2. Bend your right knee, grasp behind your thigh just above your knee in a hugging motion, and pull toward your chest. Keep your head on the floor throughout the stretch.

3. Keep your left leg slightly bent, and hold for 15 seconds.

4. Return your right leg to the floor, and repeat with your left leg.

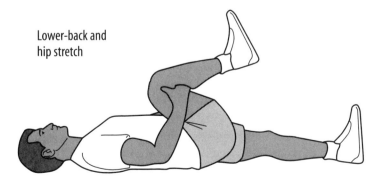

Lower-back and
hip stretch

9. Lying Hip Twist and Gluteal Stretch

PROCEDURE:

1. Lie on your back with your legs straight. Extend your arms straight out from your shoulders for balance.

2. Do not turn your head during this stretch.

3. Cross your left leg over your right leg so that your left heel is next to your right ankle. For some people, this is as far as a safe stretch should go.

4. Slowly bend your left knee, and allow the heel to slide up your right leg as far as possible. Allow your trunk to twist, and lower your bent left leg to rest on the floor. Your right hand can press gently downward on your thigh to extend the stretch. Hold for 15 seconds.

5. Slide your left leg back to the starting position, and repeat for your other side.

   Note: Your left shoulder will probably leave the floor during this stretch.

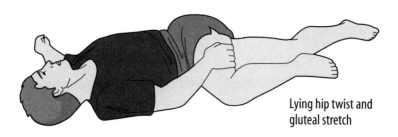

Lying hip twist and gluteal stretch

10. Groin Stretch

PROCEDURE:

1. Sit with the soles of your feet together and your knees pointing out.

2. Hold your ankles (not your toes), and slowly bring your heels toward your body.

3. While pressing down with your elbows on your thighs, bend from your hips as if to bring your chest to your feet, keeping your back straight. Hold for 15 seconds.

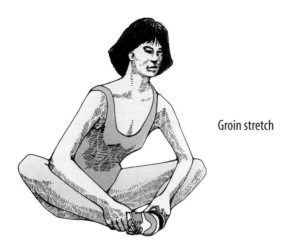

Groin stretch

᠅人 11. Hip Flexor Stretch

PROCEDURE:

1. Bend your knees, and place both hands on either side of your feet.
2. Extend your right leg behind you as far as possible, resting on your toes.
3. Keep your left knee directly above your left heel.
4. Lower the front of your pelvis toward the ground (don't expect it to move very far downward), and hold for 15 seconds.
5. Support yourself with your hands on the floor as you switch legs and repeat on your left side.

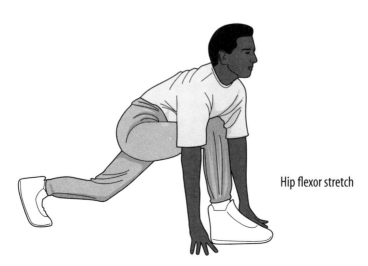

Hip flexor stretch

12. Standing Quadriceps Stretch

PROCEDURE:

1. Stand on your left leg, holding onto the wall or some other support with your left hand.
2. Bend your right knee, and grasp your right ankle with your right hand, keeping your knee pointing down.
3. Bring your right heel toward your buttocks, maintaining a wide angle between your lower and upper leg to prevent knee pain.
4. Move your right thigh directly backwards, maintaining a straight spine. Hold for 15 seconds.
5. Repeat with your left thigh.

   Note: This exercise can also be done lying on your side if no support is available or if balance is a problem.

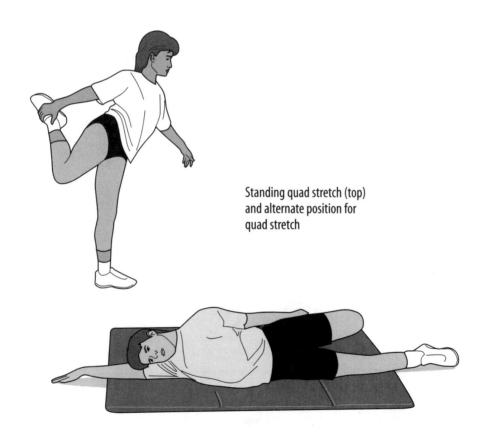

Standing quad stretch (top)
and alternate position for
quad stretch

13. Hamstring Stretch

PROCEDURE:

1. Sit on the floor with your right leg extended in front and your left leg bent at the knee so that the sole of your foot touches the inside of your right leg.
2. Keep your right kneecap facing the ceiling, and flex your foot so that your toes point straight up. Maintain this position throughout the stretch.
3. Keep your hands on the floor beside your hips throughout the stretch.
4. Arch your lower back slightly (unless painful), and lean forward from hips. Hold for 15 seconds.
5. Repeat with your left leg extended.

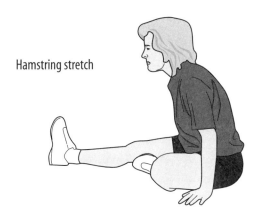

Hamstring stretch

14. Shin Stretch

PROCEDURE:

1. Stand on your left leg, supporting yourself on a chair or your thigh.
2. Slide your right foot with the top of your foot facing the ground as far behind you as possible.
3. Gently bend both knees, and lower the top of your right foot downward. Hold for 15 seconds.
4. Repeat with your left leg.
   Note: This stretch works best without shoes.

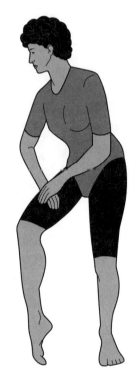

Shin stretch

⁑ㅅ 15. Calf and Achilles Tendon Stretch

PROCEDURE:

1. Stand approximately 2 feet away from a solid support (wall or tree), and place your hands at shoulder level with your arms outstretched.

2. Keep both feet facing forward throughout the stretch.

3. Extend your straight right leg back as far as possible while keeping the heel on the ground.

4. Bend your left leg to allow for a maximum stretch, and hold for 15 seconds.

5. To increase the stretch of the Achilles tendon, bring your right foot forward until your toes are next to your left heel.

6. Bend both legs and lower your body, keeping your heels on the ground. Hold for 15 seconds.

7. Switch legs, and repeat both stretches for your left leg.

   Note: This stretch can also be performed by placing your hands on your front thigh (not kneecap) for support.

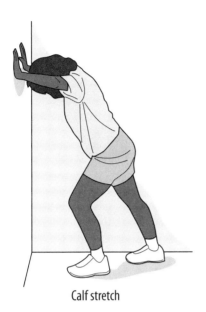

Calf stretch

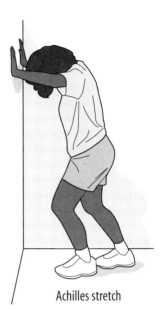

Achilles stretch

Summary

Simple stretching exercises are a sound basis for improving and maintaining flexibility. Once you learn the correct methods for performing these stretches, you can use them to increase your range of motion and allow your body to relax more fully. In turn, all physical movement becomes more comfortable and efficient.

Remember to begin each workout with some rythmical, low-intensity activity such as walking or jogging to elevate your heart and breathing rates. After this warm-up, you can perform stretches for all the muscle groups or only for those that remain particularly tight. Stretch between sets of muscular strength and endurance exercises for increased comfort and as a time-saver. After you cool down from your cardiorespiratory endurance workout, focus on stretching all the major muscle groups. Flexibility is enhanced at this time because your muscles and connective tissues are more pliable and thus responsive to stretching. Combining stretching with all the other physical fitness components will help you create a complete and highly effective fitness program.

Key Words

BALLISTIC STRETCHING: A technique for increasing flexibility that involves bouncing and momentum; generally not recommended for the average fitness participant.

FLEXIBILITY: The ability to move a joint through its full range of motion.

MINI WARM-UP: The additional period of light exercise needed to gradually increase heart and breathing rates and muscle temperature if an exerciser has stopped to stretch after an initial cardiorespiratory endurance exercise warm-up.

STATIC STRETCHING: A technique for increasing flexibility that involves holding a position at the point of slight discomfort without using bouncing or jerking motions.

A Way of Life Library

Alter, M. J. *Facilitated Stretching.* Champaign, IL: Human Kinetics, 1993.

Alter, M. J. *Science of Flexibility and Stretching.* Champaign, IL: Human Kinetics, 1996.

Alter, M. J. *Sport Stretch.* Champaign, IL: Human Kinetics, 1990.

CHAPTER 9

Advanced Fitness and Training

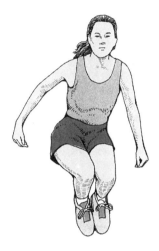

This chapter focuses on some conditioning activities that are more advanced than those discussed in previous chapters. Specifically interval training and plyometrics are forms of training normally engaged in by people who have gotten in shape and now wish to try some variations in their workouts and possibly reach a higher level of fitness.

As you read this chapter, keep these statements in mind:

• Interval training involves heavy exercise for a given distance or specified time alternated with lighter periods of exercise or rest. It differs from the run-walk technique in that the heavy exercise is performed at near maximal levels rather than at 50 to 85 percent HR reserve.

• As a general rule, the beneficial effects of various endurance-type exercise programs is the same when the total work output performed is the same. However, if you are training for sports that require quick and sudden bursts of movement, you should consider training activities that train the specific muscles involved in these activities.

• Programs that combine speed and strength training help you improve your explosiveness, a key to enhancing athletic performance.

• More and more people are participating in road races, swimming and cycling events, and multisport competitions. Preparing for such activities requires some special training considerations.

• The fitness programs described in previous chapters aimed at a level of intensity that is vigorous but well short of high-intensity training. All cardiorespiratory endurance, muscular strength and endurance, and flexibility exercises may be used as a foundation for sports participation or for more intense training.

WAY OF LIFE
Factors Influencing Interval Training Intensity

- Speed
- Length of the rest interval
- Number of work intervals
- Distance covered in each work interval

This chapter will teach you how to intensify your training and possibly help you prepare for competitive events. The key is to systematically expose your body to gradually increasing amounts of exercise. The same training principles discussed previously still apply, but now we are assuming that you are physically active and looking for an additional challenge. Continuous training, interval training, circuit training, and speed and explosiveness training can all take you to a higher state of fitness if you so desire.

Interval Training

Interval training involves bouts of exercise for a given distance or a specified time alternated with periods of recovery. As exercise tolerance permits, the speed of the exercise or the distance covered is increased gradually in succeeding workouts. Interval training differs from beginning cardiorespiratory endurance programs in that the exercise bouts are performed at near maximal levels of intensity. In other words, the heart rates and energy requirements are greater. Higher levels of discomfort are associated with this type of training, primarily because of the all-out effort that characterizes this approach. The discomfort associated with such training often stems from the increased amounts of lactic acid (a metabolic waste product) that is produced and accumulates in the muscles.

Interval training can be used with any form of cardiorespiratory endurance exercise. The intensity of interval training can be enhanced by (1) increasing the speed, (2) decreasing the rest interval, (3) increasing the number of work intervals, or (4) increasing the distance of each work interval. Changing any one or all of these factors can increase your exercise work load.

Setting Up an Interval Training Program

We will use running as the mode of exercise to show you how to set up an interval training program. Keep in mind that these same principles can apply to interval training for biking, swimming, cross-country skiing, and other cardiorespiratory endurance activities. Your exercise work load is determined from your present fitness level and your ability to recuperate after each run interval. Generally an interval program that emphasizes repetitions or distance rather than speed is better for beginners. However, for experienced runners or those who wish to improve their running speed, rigid control of the speeds of the runs and the length of the rest intervals is needed. Training of this type requires a motivated runner who will accept the challenge of the stopwatch and who can tolerate physical discomfort.

In general, the intensity of the exercise bouts should produce near maximal pulse rates. During the recovery interval, you can allow your pulse rate to slow to the lower end of your target heart rate range (that is, 50 percent) before you repeat the exercise bout. This procedure will greatly increase both cardiorespiratory endurance and muscular endurance.

TABLE 9.1
Interval Running Program

Run Time for 1.5 Miles (minutes:seconds)	Training Pace for 220 Yards/200 Meters (seconds)	Training Pace for 440 Yards/400 Meters (seconds)
8:00–8:29	37–39	74–78
8:30– 8:59	40–41	79–83
9:00–9:29	42–43	84–88
9:30–9:59	45–46	89–93
10:00–10:29	47–49	94–98
10:30–10:59	50–51	99–103
11:00–11:29	52–54	104–108
11:30–11:59	55–56	109–113
12:00–12:29	57–59	114–118
12:30–12:59	60–61	119–123
13:00–13:29	62–64	124–128
13:30–13:59	65–66	129–133
14:00–14:29	67–69	134–138
14:30–14:59	70–71	139–143
15:00–15:29	72–74	144–148
15:30–15:59	75–76	149–153
16:00 or more	77+	154+

Repetitions:
   For 220-yard runs, do 12 to 16 repetitions with a 30- to 45-second rest interval between each run.*
   For 440-yard runs, do 6 to 8 repetitions, with a 45- to 60-second rest interval between each run.*

*The time of the rest interval will depend on your pulse rate recovery.

Table 9.1 lists suggested training pace times for improving your time to run 1.5 miles. Remember, individual differences may require some modifications such as shorter or longer rest intervals, fewer or more repetitions, or varying distances run. Let's say you run 1.5 miles in 13 minutes. This means that if you ran the distance at a steady pace, you would average about 65 seconds for each 220 yards (approximately 200 meters). Your goal may be to run the 1.5-mile distance in under 12 minutes, an average of 60 seconds or less per 220 yards. To determine your training pace to achieve this goal, locate the 13:00–13:29 line in column 1 and read across to column 2 to find a recommended pace of 62 to 64 seconds for a 220-yard distance. Note that this pace is slightly faster than you can currently maintain for 1.5 miles. You need to work out at a running pace slightly faster than your best time for that particular distance. Merely running your intervals at 3 to 6 seconds faster than your best average pace will provide you with reasonable improvement. The distance of each run, the length of the rest interval between runs, and the pace are generally kept constant. It should be noted that keeping the pace constant becomes increasingly difficult as you progress through the assigned number of intervals. Including interval training workouts twice a week should be enough to help you improve your running performance. Just remember to build up gradually. Once you can handle the 62-second-pace workouts, decrease your 220-yard pace another 2 or 3 seconds to 59 or 60 seconds. In a few weeks, you will reach your goal. The same principle for regulating your training bouts can be applied to all other cardiorespiratory activities. The key is to make the pace of the work intervals slightly faster than the average pace of your best performance times.

Training for Speed and Explosiveness

Although strength is important for success in sports, speed and explosiveness are even more so. However, you need a strength base before you can develop speed and explosiveness. Recently training programs have included exercises that combine speed and strength to produce an explosive-reactive training effect. The term **plyometrics** has been used to describe these exercises. Plyometrics is a collection of jumps, hops, leaps, bounds, and skips performed at high intensity to generate the greatest amount of force in the shortest amount of time. Many coaches regard plyometrics as the key link between strength and speed. When properly practiced, plyometrics will increase your **explosiveness,** defined as the muscle's ability to generate strength as quickly and as forcefully as possible. Plyometrics bridges the gap between pure strength training and the specific skills used in competition.

The plyometric and speed exercises discussed here can enhance your athletic performance. They can help you to perform more powerfully, and they can aid in preventing injury. Because of the movements involved, plyometrics overloads muscles in a different manner from weight training. These exercises train the muscles involved to instantly recruit as many muscle fibers as possible. Maximal effort is required on each push-off, with emphasis on rebounding quickly; a minimum of time is spent on the ground. The term "touch and go" is used to describe this quick rebounding movement. Think of plyometrics as putting to work the specific strength that resistance training creates. You convert strength into explosive reactions with the ground.

Keep in mind that these exercises can be difficult to learn, exhausting to perform, and quite stressful on the body. Plyometric training is not recommended for individuals who are out of shape. If you have just started your fitness program or are resuming exercise after an extended time off (say, more than six months), follow the guidelines for cardiorespiratory (see Chapters 5 and 6) and resistance training (see Chapter 7) for at least 12 weeks prior to engaging in any formalized plyometric training program.

Plyometric training exercises take advantage of the prestretch on a muscle before you make a forceful contraction. In most physical movements, you stretch a muscle in the opposite direction just before it contracts. This causes a reflex action. This reflexive muscle contraction is more powerful than the contraction of a non-prestretched muscle. Think of the prestretch as a cocking motion. When you jump, you prestretch your thigh and leg muscles before you take off. The emphasis in plyometrics is on developing a shorter ground time when you jump, run, hop, or leap. Athletes with good strength and well-developed explosive reactions will perform better and require less time on the ground to apply the same force. Thus many runners and other athletes include some plyometric exercises and speed training in their training programs.

The following exercises are based on some basic speed and explosiveness movements used by Greg Brittenham, the strength and conditioning coach for the New York Knicks basketball team. He has used these drills with professional and amateur athletes in all sports. These drills will help you get started in a program that will enable you to become a better performer, whatever your sport or activity. But you should attempt these exercises only if you already exercise and stretch regularly, have established a muscular strength and endurance training program, and have a good cardiorespiratory base. These drills are not appropriate for someone beginning a fitness program.

1. High-Knee Marching

TECHNIQUE TIPS:
1. Use a slow tempo (approximately one step per second).
2. Focus on technique: knee lifts and arm movements.

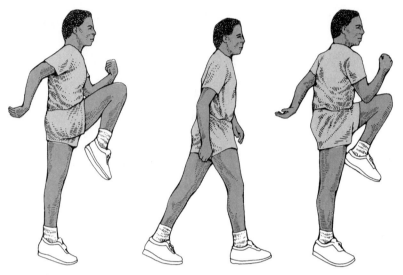

High-knee marching

3. March straight ahead, lifting your knees so that your thighs are parallel to the ground or higher.

4. Move your arms and legs in opposition (for example, left knee and right arm up).

5. Keep your supporting leg in contact with the ground; don' t skip.

2. Heel Kicks

TECHNIQUE TIPS:

1. Kick your heels up to your buttocks.

2. Point your knees toward the ground; do not lift your knees.

3. Point your toes toward the sky as your heels graze your buttocks.

3. High-Knee Run

TECHNIQUE TIPS:

1. Run straight ahead, lifting your knees so that your thighs are parallel to the ground or higher.

2. Move your arms and legs in opposition (for example, left knee and right arm up).

3. Use a tempo similar to running.

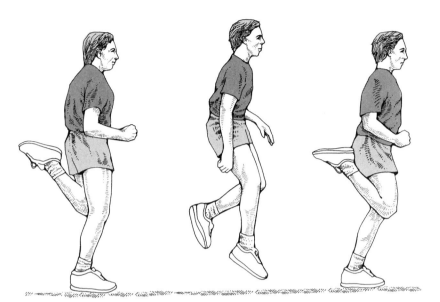

Heel kicks

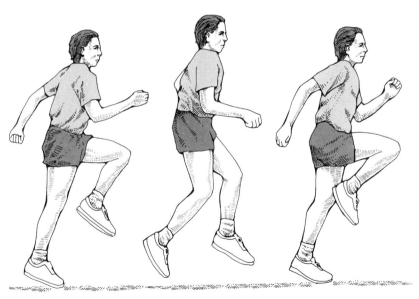

High-knee run

🏃 *4. High-Knee Skipping for Flexibility*

TECHNIQUE TIPS:

1. Skip, alternating legs.
2. Drive with knees high.
3. Use high opposite-arm action.
4. Extend your drive leg, with your foot leaving the ground in a skipping motion.

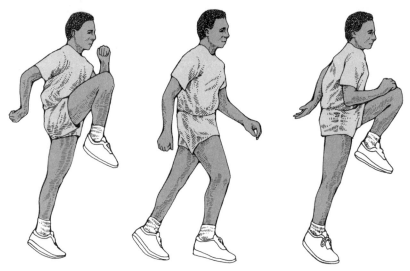

High-knee skipping for flexibility

🏃 *5. High-Knee Skipping for Power*

TECHNIQUE TIPS:

1. Skip, alternating legs.
2. Use a more forceful arm and leg drive (for longer, higher skips).
3. Minimize your time on the ground.

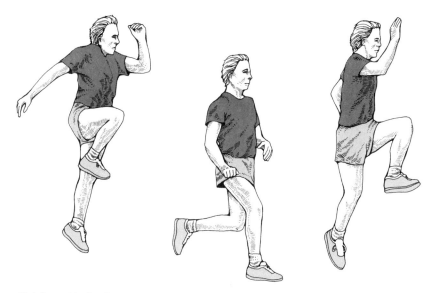

High-knee skipping for power

:ᐟ 6. High-Knee Fast-Frequency Sprint

TECHNIQUE TIPS:

1. Establish a fast-frequency run similar to the high-knee run.
2. Maintain the frequency as you lengthen your stride.

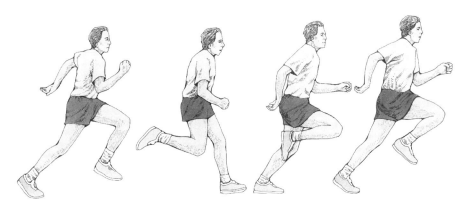

High-knee fast-frequency sprint

7. Vertical Jumps

TECHNIQUE TIPS:

1. Jump from a standing position to touch a basketball backboard.
2. Alternate hands.
3. Emphasize a quick "touch and go" as your toes touch the floor.

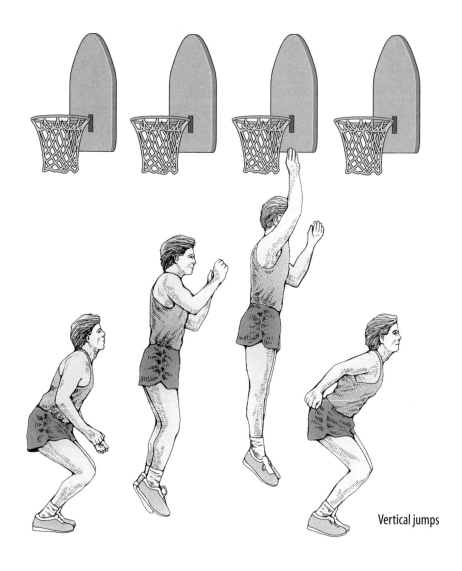

Vertical jumps

⛹ 8. Standing Long Jump

TECHNIQUE TIPS:

1. Prestretch your arms and back.
2. Prestretch your thighs and legs.
3. Jump out and away.

Standing long jumps

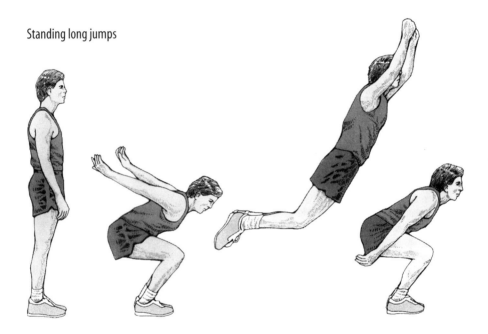

⛹ 9. Quick-Response Jumps (Double Leg)

TECHNIQUE TIPS:

1. Jump as high as possible moving forward slowly.
2. Do not bend your knees.
3. Stay on the balls of your feet.
4. Keep in mind that if you can jump as much as 3 inches off the ground, you are doing exceptionally well.

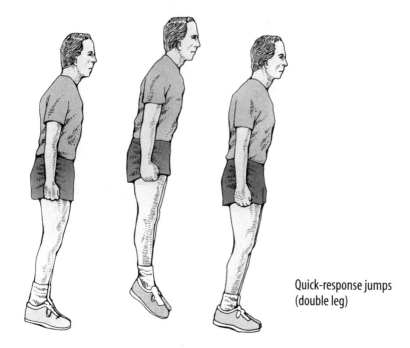

Quick-response jumps
(double leg)

10. Small Barrier Jumps

TECHNIQUE TIPS:

1. Keep your feet together.
2. Concentrate on getting off the ground quickly.
3. Jump from side to side.
4. Do a separate set jumping from front to back.

W A Y   O F   L I F E
Plyometrics Checklist

- Perform on a carpeted or matted surface, not on a hard floor.
- Rest at least two days between workouts.

- Begin with low-intensity marches, skips, hops, and drops.
- Perform plyometrics before other strength and conditioning exercises.

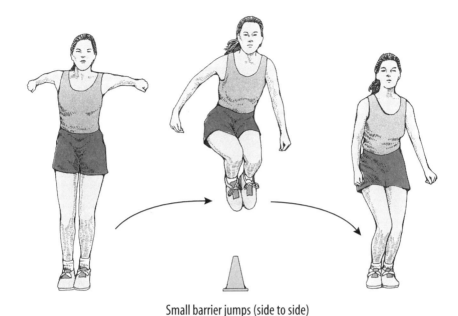

Small barrier jumps (side to side)

These drills can be incorporated into your regular physical fitness training. However, power development drills need only be performed once or twice a week. Start out with marching, heel kicks, and high-knee skipping for flexibility. You need to do only three sets of each drill (a set refers to 10 to 12 foot contacts as counted for one foot). Be sure to rest for at least 30 seconds between sets. As your body becomes accustomed to the vigorous impact, you can add drills such as the high-knee fast-frequency sprint and the jumps. Keep in mind that although this is only a start-up program, it can still help you to perform more explosively.

Fitness Events

What Are Your Opportunities?

People who get themselves into good physical condition often become involved in some form of competition such as running and cycling road races or swimming events. At this point, you may be quite content with your fitness workouts. Being in shape is a satisfying feeling. However, more often than not, once you reach this level of physiological fitness, you may be wondering what it would be like to participate in a local "fun run." We encourage you to participate and enjoy the fellowship. The aim is not so much to compete against people, but rather to participate with peers who are all into the same mind-set of being physically fit. Local 5-kilometer (approximately 3 miles) or 10-kilometer (approximately 6.2 miles) runs are excellent events in which to test yourself. For many people, setting goals throughout the year to participate in such events also helps to maintain motivation during workouts.

Increasing numbers of people also are participating in multisport competitions. These contests generally feature a combination of two or more endurance-type activities, such as a distance run combined with cycling and swimming events. These events often are referred to as **triathlons.** Cross-country skiing, horseback riding, kayaking, and canoeing are other activities that might be included in a multisport event. These rugged contests call for continuous exertion, and the objective is to endure rather than race against the clock. For example, a typical event might include a 1-mile swim in a lake, an 18-mile bike ride, and a 6-mile run (footrace). There are many variations of the triathlon, the most famous and toughest being the Iron Man Triathlon, staged each year in Hawaii. This grueling event features a 2.4-mile ocean swim, a 112-mile bike ride, and a 26.2-mile **marathon.** However, most triathlons involve more moderate distances.

The growth of multisport events has been quite rapid. According to *Triathlon Today,* a multisport publication, close to 1,000 triathlon events are held in the United States each year. When you include biathlons (two-sport events), the number of multisport events is around 1,500. Some events are even held inside where facilities permit. Triathlons are a natural extension of the fitness and running movement that has blossomed over the last two decades. These events represent a branching-out to a variety of worthy fitness activities.

Training Suggestions for Fitness Events

Here are some suggestions for training that will help you to participate in some of the many competitive activities that are available. Many of us lack the genetic endowment to become outstanding runners, cyclists, swimmers, or other types of athletes. Nevertheless, adherence to certain training guidelines can assist you in performing at or near your physical potential. Whether you enter a hometown 10K run or the New York Marathon, preparing for and participating in such events can be quite satisfying.

Before entering an event such as a running race, you should be able to cover the designated distance during your training in your target heart-rate range. During the event, you will probably run at a much higher intensity (85 to 90 percent HR reserve). It does take some long-range planning to prepare properly and avoid injury. Figure 9.1 shows a training program for a **half-marathon** (13.1 miles) that has been effective for people running their first half-marathon. It is assumed that you can easily run 3 to 4 miles four days a

FIGURE 9.1
A Half-Marathon Training Program (miles per day and week)

Week	Sun.	Mon.	Tues.	Wed.	Thurs.	Fri.	Sat.	Total
1	3		3	2	3		3	14
2	3		4	3	3		3	16
3	4		4	3	4		3	18
4	4		4	4	4		4	20
5	5		4	5	4		4	22
6	6		5	4	5		4	24
7	8		5	4	5		4	26
8	8		6	4	6		4	28
9	8		6	5	6		5	30
10	10		6	5	6		5	32
11	12		6	5	6		5	34
12	10		6	5	6		5	32
13	12		6	5	6		5	34
14	10		6	5	8		5	34
15	7		4	3			13.1	27.1

week before engaging in this training regimen. Note that you increase your total running distance 2 miles each week. Also the program is timed so that you can run 10 to 12 miles one month before the event. A basic rule is that you should be able to cover 75 to 90 percent of the distance of the event at least one month prior. This assures a good training base.

Most endurance-type training involves three phases. In phase 1, you increase your average daily mileage. In phase 2, you level out and adapt to this increased level of training. In phase 3, you taper off your training by reducing your mileage about a week before the race so you are well rested for the actual competition.

Although you want to progressively increase your mileage, you also need to pay attention to the type of mileage you run each week. Some of your weekly mileage (25 percent or so) should be at a pace faster than your target heart rate. If you are going to run long distances (such as half-marathons or full marathons), then you should cover about one-fourth of your weekly mileage during one of your workouts. For example, if you are up to 50 miles a week, then one workout should be 12 to 13 miles. Also, you should alternate a hard day of training with an easy day. Fortunately your body has an uncanny ability to adapt to this stress when given a proper recovery period, thus reaching a higher exercise tolerance. And don't overlook the importance of a rest day. Along with alternating several hard training days with several easy workout days, you should allow at least one day a week to rest your body.

To increase your mileage safely, up your weekly total by no more than 10 percent a week. About every fourth week of training, you may want to reduce your mileage to 80 percent of the previous week's total. Then increase your mileage back to the previous week's total and, if you wish, continue on a progressive 10 percent mileage increase per week.

Do not run the same distance each day. You should vary not only your distances but also the speed at which you run (or cycle or swim). One way to do this is to incorporate interval training into one of your workouts. A danger in interval training is the risk for injury. However, if you wish to increase your running or cycling time and have the ability to do so, then you should include some shorter bouts at a quicker pace and a higher intensity. In the case of running, such exercise bouts could consist of a relatively short 440-yard run or a 1-mile run with walking or light running in between the runs. The key is to find what suits you.

Uphill training can also be a vital component of your total program. Hill running helps you develop good quadriceps endurance. If you are going to run a race with hills, then you definitely need to practice hill running—both up and down. Hill running lets you experience some pain and fatigue similar to that encountered in a racing situation; moreover, it helps you develop a psychological toughness that is important in competition. This type of training for competition (whether in running, cycling, or swimming) is not exactly a fun activity. The fun comes later, when you have successfully completed the event.

Training for a long run such as the 26.2-mile marathon requires some careful planning. Prospective participants need a three- to four-month period of training to get to the point where they can complete a training run of 18 to 21 miles four to five weeks prior to the marathon. It is generally not necessary to cover the total 26.2-mile distance before you run the actual marathon. During your long training runs, you need to practice drinking water every few miles to become accustomed to taking in fluids. Fluid replacement is a must for anyone participating in a long-distance running or cycling event. In general, you need to complete a couple of 20-mile-or-more runs four to six weeks prior to the actual marathon to safely run the 26.2-mile distance and avoid injury. Many people enter these events improperly prepared and experience injury and body regulation problems as a result. Approximately 8 to 10 days prior to the marathon, you should be able to run 14 to 16 miles with ease and recover comfortably within about an hour after the run. If you don't respond in this manner, then you may not be adequately prepared for the event.

Keep in mind that successful training is as much a function of the head as of the body. Some of the suggestions given here may seem quite conservative. However, you must always train well within your capabilities, gradually building up mileage and, in some cases, speed. Being able to handle the increased distance is most important. Trying to increase your weekly distance too rapidly can result in injury. Training for a triathlon requires application of the same principles for each of the three activities. Thus such training requires more time.

Remember, you don't need to go all out each day. Establish a sensible goal that suits you. If you adhere to the guidelines presented in this chapter, then you will be ready for the fun of reaching your goal. And regardless of where you finish, recognize that all finishers are winners.

Summary

Competition is a way of life. Consider your preparation and training for an event as a journey. If you maintain the proper perspective, your training program can be a fun and interesting challenge. It may also provide the incentive for staying in shape. For many people, the competition itself is not so important. To them, the training becomes a form of social involvement and an enjoyable way to become and keep fit. You should not put too much emphasis on the competitive aspects of your exercise program. You could feel frustrated, you could overextend yourself, and you could defeat the real purpose of your program. Setting reasonable goals as you extend yourself physically can add interest to your quest to be physically fit. Compete only with yourself, and set goals that you can reach. Success and improvement are great motivators that can reinforce your exercise program. Regular training with periodic participation in competitions such as fun runs, bike tours, triathlons, racquetball tournaments, and cross-country ski events can be rewarding. Such recreational events will help you to realize the pleasures of being active and feeling good about yourself. Most important, participating with friends, whether in preparation for or during an event, may be the most fulfilling part of the process.

Key Words

EXPLOSIVENESS: A muscle's ability to generate force as quickly as possible.

HALF-MARATHON: A footrace of 13.1 miles, half the distance of a marathon.

INTERVAL TRAINING: Training made up of successive bouts of exercise at near maximal intensity alternated with periods of rest or lighter exercise such as brisk walking or slow jogging.

MARATHON: A footrace covering 26.2 miles.

PLYOMETRICS: Exercises designed to improve one's muscle power or explosiveness.

TRIATHLON: A competitive event involving three endurance-type activities such as swimming, cycling, and running.

A Way of Life Library

Brittenham, D., and G. Brittenham. *Stronger Abs and Back.* Champaign, IL: Human Kinetics, 1997.

Brittenham, G. *Complete Conditioning for Basketball.* Champaign, IL: Human Kinetics, 1996.

Chu, D. A. *Jumping into Plyometrics.* Champaign, IL: Human Kinetics, 1993.

Chu, D. A. *Explosive Power and Strength.* Champaign, IL: Human Kinetics, 1996.

Wilmore, J. H., and D. L. Costill. *Physiology of Sport and Exercise.* Champaign, IL: Human Kinetics, 1994.

CHAPTER **10**

Nutrition and Exercise

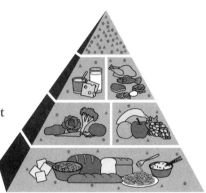

Nutrition relates to what foods we eat and how our bodies process them. Now that you understand how to develop and follow a sound exercise program, you're ready to adopt good eating habits, which will make it even easier to reach your fitness and health goals. In this chapter, we discuss basic nutrition facts to help you make sensible decisions that will positively affect your physical performance.

Weight management, or more specifically, management of body composition, is possible when energy intake from nutrients is closely balanced with the energy expended during work, play, and rest. Small increases in intake or expenditure can cause controllable increases in weight gain or loss, respectively. Much has been written about innumerable diets and weight loss programs. Unfortunately much of this information lacks a sound scientific basis. This chapter focuses on how regular vigorous exercise combined with a sensible eating plan can effectively control body composition. In addition, we discuss common misconceptions about exercise and fat control and present approximate energy costs for a variety of physical activities.

As you read this chapter, keep these statements in mind:

- Managing body composition requires a knowledge of energy intake (food) and energy output (physical activity).
- Proteins are the basic structural substance of the body; carbohydrates and fats are the primary energy sources.
- Your daily energy needs depend on such factors as your age, body size, amount of muscle mass, and the type and amount of your daily physical activity.

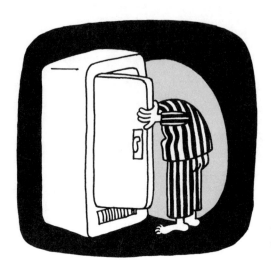

Eating for health is not about deprivation, but about moderation.

- Body composition (the proportion of fat to muscle tissue in your body) is a much more useful indicator of physical fitness and health than scale weight.
- Exercise levels can be classified from low to vigorous based on multiples of resting energy expenditure.
- Research does not support the theory that if you exercise an area of your body, you will reduce the excess fat in that region (spot reduction).
- The practice of dehydrating (losing water) is an ineffective and dangerous method of fat loss.
- Eating for health is not about deprivation or unreasonable restrictions, but about moderation.

Nutrition Basics

Foods provide us with a wide variety of essential substances, or **nutrients.** Nutrients are necessary for building and repairing the body and for providing the energy needed for efficient functioning. Energy is provided by three basic classes of nutrients: proteins, carbohydrates, and fats. Minerals, vitamins, and water are also nutrients, but they do not provide us with energy. To determine your daily requirements of nutrients, you need to know your body weight in kilograms. Because a kilogram is equal to approximately 2.2 pounds, simply divide your weight in pounds by 2.2 to convert to kilograms.

In this section, we summarize the role of each nutrient.

Proteins

Proteins are the basic structural substance of every cell in the body. Protein gives structure to bones, skin, muscle fibers, and many tissues. Whereas proteins serve as the framework, carbohydrates and fats provide the energy for the body to work and move about. Enzymes and hormones are proteins that control and regulate chemical reactions in our bodies. Specialized proteins are also present in the blood in the form of clotting agents and oxygen-carrying molecules. Proteins are not significant sources of energy during physical activity unless that activity is of very long duration, such as an ultramarathon, or unless you have an extremely poor diet.

The protein we eat is broken down into basic building blocks called **amino acids.** The amino acids are then put back together in various parts of the body to form structural proteins and enzymes. Major sources of complete proteins come from foods of animal origin: meat, fish, poultry, eggs, and milk. Unfortunately protein-rich foods from animal sources are generally high in fat as well. Luckily there are excellent low-fat versions of these foods such as skim milk, low-fat yogurts, reduced-fat cheeses, lean meats, and some skinless poultry. Also, specific combinations of lower-fat nonanimal proteins such as peas, beans, and grains can provide all the necessary amino acids in your diet.

Fifteen percent of your total calories should come from protein. One gram of protein equals 4 calories. To calculate the number of protein calories in your food, simply multiply the number of protein grams by 4. If you don't want to count calories, multiply your body weight in kilograms by 0.8 to get the number of grams of protein needed per day.

Carbohydrates

Carbohydrates provide us with energy for performing bodily functions, such as forming new chemical compounds, transmitting nerve impulses, and supplying the primary energy for vigorous muscular activity. The carbohydrates we eat are broken down to provide **glucose.** The glucose then enters the bloodstream as **blood sugar,** which is used for energy or stored in the liver and other cells as **glycogen.**

There are many forms of carbohydrates, such as lactose (a sugar found in milk), fructose (a fruit sugar), fiber, and starches. Beneficial sources of carbohydrates include fruits and vegetables and their pure extracted juices. Equally important starch sources include potatoes, rice, peas, whole grain cereals (such as wheat, oats, corn, and rice), pasta, bread, and bagels.

Carbohydrate foods like candy, jams, jellies, table sugar, honey, molasses, and concentrated syrups (like corn syrup) are high in refined sugar content and are called "empty-calorie" foods because they provide energy but little or no other nutrients. Direct your focus instead on eating foods that provide a better nutrient return for the caloric investment. The consumption of refined sugars should be limited when they interfere with adequate intake of other nutrients or maintenance of proper energy balance. According to estimates, the average American consumes well over 100 pounds of refined sugar per year, and the typical American diet has 25 percent or more of its calories in the form of sugar. Much of these sugars are hidden in the processed foods that we consume regularly, such as ketchup and fruit cocktail drinks.

Approximately 55 percent of the calories you eat should come from the carbohydrates found in vegetables, fruits, and starches. The Senate Select Committee on Nutrition and Human Needs recommends cutting your intake of refined sugar (sucrose) to about 15 percent of your total calories. This means that 40 percent of your total calories should be carbohydrates other than refined sugar. Keep in mind, however, that even though complex carbohydrates are usually considered the "good guys" in the battle of the bulge, you can eat too much of a good thing. Whenever you take in more carbohydrates than your body needs, the excess is converted to fat and stored, increasing the body's fat content. Just like protein, each gram of carbohydrate equals 4 calories.

Considerable evidence suggests that refined sugars do contribute to tooth decay. Refined sugars also are frequently blamed for a number of other health problems such as diabetes, heart disease, and certain behavioral disorders. Currently there is no evidence that sugars contribute directly to these health problems. However, obesity appears to be a major determinant of diabetes, more than doubling the risk for its development for every 20 percent of excess body weight. Thus sugar may play an indirect role in the development of diabetes by contributing to excess energy intake and eventually to obesity.

Fats

Fats exist in the body primarily as **triglycerides,** which are composed of **fatty acids.** Besides being an important part of the cell structure, fat acts as an insulator and protector of vital body parts. Fat is also a major source of energy for muscular activity. Gram for gram, fats provide more than twice as much energy (9 calories per gram) as either carbohydrates or protein. Common sources of fats are meat, butter, margarine, shortening, cooking and salad oils, cream, most cheeses, mayonnaise, nuts, whole milk, eggs, and milk chocolate. Of course, anything cooked in fat will contain fat.

Not all fats are alike. There are two types of fats: **saturated** and **unsaturated.** Saturated fats come from meat, whole milk, cheese, and butter. This type of fat is generally solid at room temperature. Saturated fats and the "tropical" oils (coconut and palm) are known to raise levels of cholesterol in the bloodstream. For this reason, it is important to reduce these fats in your diet. No more than 30 percent of your daily calories should come from fat, with 10 percent or less coming from saturated fat sources. Replace as much of the saturated fat in your diet as possible with monounsaturated or polyunsaturated fats. These unsaturated fats tend to be in a liquid form at room temperature. The monounsaturated fats are found in canola, peanut, and olive oils. Polyunsaturated fats are found in corn, soybean, cottonseed, sunflower, and safflower oils.

Cholesterol, a fattylike substance, is found only in animal products, especially egg yolks, liver, and brains, and in shrimp, lobster, and other crustaceans. Cholesterol is necessary; in fact, your body is capable of producing its own cholesterol. It is required for many of the complex functions of the body and is used in making the sex hormones testosterone and estrogen. When there is too much cholesterol, however, it tends to settle in the walls of the blood vessels and can impair circulation. (For more information on cholesterol and its relationship to heart disease, see Chapter 11.)

Minerals

Minerals are essential inorganic substances that give strength to certain body tissues and assist with numerous vital functions. Calcium, iodine, iron, phosphorus, magnesium, and other minerals are vital to the functioning of the body systems. For example, calcium is the most abundant mineral in the body and combines with phosphorus to form the bones and teeth. Calcium is also crucial for normal functioning of the muscles. Phosphorus plays an essential role in supplying energy to the body. Iodine is an important ingredient in thyroxin, a hormone that governs the rate of energy metabolism in the body. Iron is a key component of hemoglobin, which enables blood to carry oxygen.

Sodium and potassium are also minerals that play a key role in controlling and regulating fluid balance in the body. These electrolytes are found mainly in the fluids inside and outside the cells and are essential for the proper transmission of nerve impulses. Sodium is present in all living matter including meat, poultry, fish, and vegetables. It is also added in the processing of food as a preservative and stabilizer and for taste (in the form of table salt). High blood pressure is related to excess amounts of salt or, more precisely, sodium in the diet. (For more information on high blood pressure, see Chapter 11.) You should limit your sodium intake by not salting food and by avoiding products containing sodium additives. A recent decision by many food companies to limit the salt in their products or even eliminate it entirely reflects the growing awareness of the harmful effects of excess salt in the diet.

Vitamins

Vitamins are organic substances that are essential for the proper functioning of muscles and nerves. They also play a dynamic role in releasing energy from foods and in promoting normal growth of body tissues. Because the cells of the body cannot form these substances, you must provide the vitamin needs of your body through your diet.

Some vitamins tend to be retained within the body and stored in fat (fat-soluble vitamins). Megadose supplements of the fat-soluble vitamins may accumulate, creating toxic conditions in the body. Many vitamins, however, are transported in the fluids of the tissues and cells and are not stored (water-soluble vitamins). Any excess amounts of the water-soluble vitamins are usually excreted in the urine on a daily basis.

Until recently, it was generally accepted that all the required vitamins could be obtained from a well-rounded, nutritious diet. However, ongoing research has focused on the contribution of certain vitamins called antioxidants and their role in retarding the destruction of our cells. In particular, vitamins E and C and beta carotene (vitamin A) are frequently taken as supplements in much higher doses than previously considered safe or necessary. For further information on antioxidants, refer to Kenneth H. Cooper's *Antioxidant Revolution* (see A Way of Life Library).

Vitamin and Mineral Supplementation

Health experts recommend that we consume three to five servings of vegetables and two to four servings of fruit daily, but the reality is that the vast majority of Americans do not. There are a variety of reasons for this. Our hectic lifestyles often do not allow for well-planned daily meals, and we do not keep track of what we eat from meal to meal. In addition, we may not care for the taste or texture of many of the healthier foods or not take the time and effort to learn to prepare them in more enticing ways. Also, some of the better sources of specific vitamins (such as vitamin E) are high in fat and calories, which many of us are trying to reduce in our diets. You would be wise to keep a three-day dietary intake record (see G. Kostas in A Way of Life Library) and consult with a registered dietitian before adding or deleting anything from your diet. Upon examination of your own diet, you may find a need for supplementation in order to ensure 100 percent of the recommended daily allowances of certain vitamins and minerals. Of course, *eating foods that contain a variety of nutrients, vitamins, and minerals is always the best option, particularly since there may be other benefits of eating whole foods that we are not aware of at this time.*

Water

Because nearly 60 to 70 percent of the human body is water, our need for water is second only to our need for oxygen. Water provides the medium (body fluids) for transporting nutrients and hormones throughout the body and for

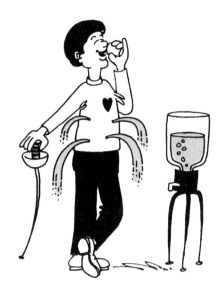

Get into the habit of drinking water frequently during your exercise sessions.

removing wastes from the body. Water also plays a vital role in regulating body temperature. You get water not only by drinking it directly but also from the foods you eat. Caffeinated beverages such as coffee, many teas, colas, and various other soft drinks act as diuretics, causing frequent urination and thus water loss. Thus, when determining whether you are ingesting enough water on a daily basis, you should not include these beverages. In fact, you need to drink additional water for every caffeinated drink to replace the water lost through urination.

Get into the habit of drinking water frequently throughout your day and particularly at regular intervals during your exercise sessions. Because dehydration can begin before you feel thirsty, do not rely on thirst to gauge your need for water. In general, drink at least eight glasses of water a day or 1 liter for every 1,000 calories you expend. When participating in vigorous exercise where sweating is constant and abundant, drink a cup of water every 15 minutes. If possible, drink cool water, as it is more easily absorbed than room-temperature water.

Guidelines for Good Nutrition

As a general rule, you can meet your daily nutritional needs by following the recommendations of the Food Guide Pyramid (see Figure 10.1). There are six groupings of food choices in the pyramid, not the famous four food groups of the past. The pyramid more thoroughly breaks down the food choice categories and does not treat all choices as nutritionally equal. Serving suggestions give a range to guide the smaller person (lower number) as well as the larger person (higher number) in deciding how many servings to eat from each group. Perhaps the pyramid's greatest contribution is its symbolic depiction of the food groups that should be most abundant in our diets (those at or near the base) versus those that should be eaten sparingly (those at or near the tip). You will also find the Food Guide Pyramid imprinted on many packaged foods.

After studying the Food Guide Pyramid and evaluating your daily food selections, you may find that some adjustments are in order. For example, you may be eating the right foods but in the wrong balance. Instead of building your evening meal around meat, you might make your meat a side dish with pasta and vegetables as the main course. Healthy eating focuses on a reduction of fats, moderate protein intake, and increased consumption of complex carbohydrates rather than sugary foods and drinks. Remember, many bakery goods such as cookies, pastries, and pies tend to contain high levels of fat and sugar. For example, 50 percent of the total caloric value of some cookies comes from fat. A simple way to tell if a food is low in fat (30 percent or less) is to check the nutrition label on the packaging. Either calories from fat, percentage fat, or grams of fat will be listed. Remember, fat contains 9 calories per gram, so choose foods with no more than 3 fat grams per 100 calories (3 gm $\times$ 9 cals = 27 fat cals, or less than 30 percent fat). If you yearn for baked goods, make your own low-fat versions by substituting applesauce (or other pureed fruits) for oil and using egg whites instead of whole eggs in the recipes. You will be pleasantly surprised at the good taste and the drastic reduction in fat content.

Specific Recommendations

Health organizations, the federal government, and scientific groups have responded to the demand for simple and safe nutritional guidelines by publishing recommendations directed at healthy North American adults and children. Following are some of these guidelines. Keep in mind that research seems to bring forth nutritional breakthroughs almost monthly and that remaining informed is important in these ever-changing times. These dietary guidelines are hardly revolutionary. Many nutrition experts have been making these recommendations for years. At first, the meat, dairy, and egg industries criticized these suggestions as unproven. However, these industries are now researching ways to make their products more healthful.

1. *Reduce total fat intake to 30 percent or less of your total calories, and reduce saturated fats to less than one-third of your total fat intake.* Diets low in saturated fats are associated with low rates of heart disease and related cardiovascular ailments. By substituting fish, skinless poultry, lean meats, and

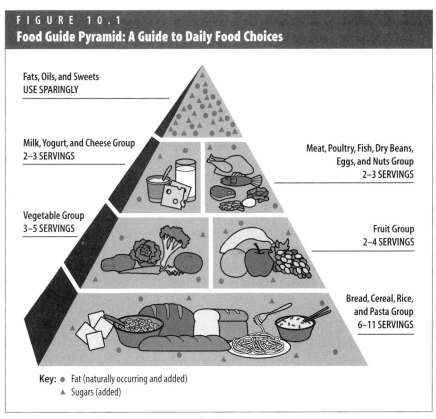

FIGURE 10.1
Food Guide Pyramid: A Guide to Daily Food Choices

Fats, Oils, and Sweets
USE SPARINGLY

Milk, Yogurt, and Cheese Group
2–3 SERVINGS

Meat, Poultry, Fish, Dry Beans,
Eggs, and Nuts Group
2–3 SERVINGS

Vegetable Group
3–5 SERVINGS

Fruit Group
2–4 SERVINGS

Bread, Cereal, Rice,
and Pasta Group
6–11 SERVINGS

Key: ● Fat (naturally occurring and added)
▲ Sugars (added)

Source: U.S. Department of Agriculture, U.S. Department of Health and Human Services.

low-fat or nonfat dairy products, you can lower your total fat intake without giving up the iron and calcium these foods provide. Limit your intake of fried foods, baked goods (those that contain high levels of fat), spreads (for example, butter), and dressings containing fats and oils. Replacing these fats with monounsaturated fats such as olive oil and canola oil has been shown to be very beneficial. Omega-6 and omega-3 polyunsaturated fats are recommended. Omega-3 oils are found in fish such as salmon and mackerel and in some plant oils. Omega-6 oils are common in such plant oils as corn, soybean, safflower, and sunflower.

2. *Reduce intake of cholesterol to less than 300 milligrams (mg) daily.* Organ meats, some shellfish, and egg yolks are all high in cholesterol and should be limited. In addition, the main sources of cholesterol-raising saturated fats are high-fat dairy and meat products.

3. *Eat the Food Guide Pyramid's recommended servings of vegetables and fruits every day, and increase your intake of starches and other complex carbohydrates by combining six or more servings of breads, cereals, and legumes.* Pay particular attention to increasing servings of green and yellow vegetables and citrus fruits. A serving is equal to a half cup of fresh or cooked vegetables, fruits, or cereal. A slice of bread, a roll, and a medium-size piece of fruit also represent an average serving. Carbohydrates, especially complex carbohydrates (such as are found in potatoes, breads, vegetables, and fruits), are all good substitutes for fatty foods and good sources of several vitamins and minerals and of fiber.

4. *Maintain protein intake at moderate levels.* Earlier you learned that protein is an essential nutrient, providing the structure in all cells of the body. The recommended dietary allowance (RDA) for protein each day is 0.8 grams (g) per kilogram (kg) of your body weight. However, studies have revealed that the average protein intake in the typical American diet for adults is considerably higher than the RDA. There are no known benefits and possibly some risks from eating high levels of animal protein. Once again, you do not need to eliminate meat from your diet. Simply eat lean meat, which is low in saturated fat, in smaller portions. An easy way to determine your meat portion is to make it no larger than the size of your clenched fist.

5. *Balance food intake and physical activity to maintain appropriate body composition.* Extreme restriction of food intake, such as through fasting and very low-calorie diets, is dangerous. Managing your body composition is infinitely easier when you combine good nutrition with regular exercise. Today we know that excess body fat is a serious health problem that increases your risk for several chronic disorders such as adult-onset diabetes, high blood pressure, and circulatory and respiratory diseases, to name a few. Ways to manage your body fat with regular exercise will be discussed later in this chapter.

6. *Avoid alcoholic beverages.* Daily alcoholic beverage consumption should be limited to no more than two cans of beer, two small glasses of wine, or two average-size cocktails. Not only is alchohol a source of empty calories, it also interferes with your body's ability to break down and use fat. It is well established that excessive alcohol consumption increases the risk for many diseases, including heart disease, liver disease, neurological disease, and some forms of cancer, as well as many nutritional deficiencies. Additionally pregnant women should avoid alcoholic beverages altogether. To date, no safe level of alcohol intake during pregnancy has been established, and there is a risk of damage to the fetus with alcohol consumption.

- Eat a variety of foods.
- Maintain a healthy level of body fat.
- Choose a diet low in fat, saturated fat, and cholesterol.
- Choose a diet with plenty of vegetables, fruits, and grains.
- Use sugar in moderation.
- Restrict the use of salt and sodium.
- If you drink alcohol, do so in moderation.

Source: Nutrition and Your Health: Dietary Guidelines for Americans (Washington, DC: U.S. Department of Agriculture, U.S. Department of Health and Human Services, 1980).

7. *Limit the use of salt to a total daily intake of 6 grams or less.* Elevated blood pressure is associated with salt intake above 6 grams per day, a level that Americans habitually exceed. Nutritionists now stress that you should limit or even avoid the use of salt in cooking. And you should definitely avoid adding salt to your food at the table. Many foods, especially the readily available processed foods, are heavily salted and should be consumed sparingly.

8. *Obtain adequate calcium.* Calcium is an essential nutrient for maintaining adequate health of the bones, muscles, and teeth. Women, due to their lower caloric intake and their increased risk for osteoporosis, and young people, due to a higher nutrient requirement, need to be very selective in their food choices to obtain adequate calcium. Rich sources of calcium are low-fat or nonfat dairy products (for example., skim milk and reduced-fat cheeses) and dark-green vegetables (for example, broccoli and brussel sprouts). Calcium supplements are also popular, especially for individuals who cannot tolerate the milk sugar, lactose. A nutritionist or physician can direct your use of calcium supplementation.

Nutritional Fads and Fallacies

For centuries, people have been searching for the magic substances that would provide things like perpetual youth, optimal health, and/or athletic prowess. In this section, we discuss some common nutritional fads and fallacies. (For more in-depth reading on these topics, refer to A Way of Life Library at the end of this chapter.)

Nutritional Ergogenic Aids

Special foods or supplements that are touted to improve physical fitness levels or athletic performance are known as **nutritional ergogenic aids.** Just because a food or supplement has been labeled as a nutritional ergogenic aid does not mean its effects have been proven to improve health or athletic performance. In fact, the claims of many of the products that have been tested for ergogenic effects are unfounded. However, many manufacturers have preyed on our inherent desire for substances that will enhance health and performance. In the process, they have turned nutritional ergogenics into a multibillion-dollar industry. Although hard to swallow (no pun intended), research findings do not support the use of nutritional ergogenic aids for individuals eating a balanced diet. Table 10.1 lists some of the more popular nutritional ergogenic aids that are not necessary for the general fitness enthusiast.

Finally do not assume that the Food and Drug Administration (FDA) has approved a nutritional supplement just because it is available at your local grocery or health food store. Products classified as supplements do not need FDA approval before being sold. In fact, only if the product causes negative health side effects will the FDA step in and conduct tests. In other words, you are paying to be the guinea pig for many of these products.

The "Other White Meat"

In a quest to enhance its market share, the pork industry started an ad campaign stating that pork is the "other white meat." The not-so-hidden meaning in these ads is that pork is similar in fat composition to chicken or turkey. Do not be misled. Depending on the cut of meat, today's "leaner pork" can range from 26 to 54 percent fat calories while skinless chicken can range from 19 to 47 percent. The bottom line is, no matter what the animal source—whether poultry, beef, or pork—do your homework. Consult a nutrition book to determine the leanest cuts and ways to prepare them. Do not fall prey to advertising hype.

Liquid Boosts

Liquid diet drinks were originally developed to meet the nutritional needs of patients unable to eat or digest solid foods. Now advertisers for these liquid meals would have you believe that using these products will "boost your energy levels" or serve as food for people on the go. Yes, these drinks do supply ample calories (approximately 300 calories), but they also contain lots of sugar and more fat than you might expect. Experts emphasize that these drinks should not take the place of a balanced diet and do not add a "boost" to energy levels for those practicing good nutrition. They also stress that even the busiest of schedules allow for eating foods like fruits, yogurt, or bagels. Again, read labels, plan your snacks, and be an informed consumer.

TABLE 10.1 Substances Touted as Nutritional Ergogenic Aids	
Substance	**Description and Claims***
Bee pollen	Taken from bees or directly from plants; increases energy and vitality.
L-carnitine	Increases fat-burning capability.[†] *Note:* DL-carnitine, a different form than L-carnitine, has been shown to be toxic.
Chromium picolinate	Enhances metabolism; increases muscle mass.
Choline	Increases fat-burning capability. *Note:* This substance has been shown to cause gastric upset with mega-doses.
Ginseng	Serves as a tonic for many ailments; increases strength and aerobic capacity.
Coenzyme Q_{10} (ubiquinone)	Increases aerobic capacity[†]; improves immunity to disease.
Inosine	Increases anaerobic performance and muscle contractility. *Note:* This substance has been shown to cause gout and sore, aching joints.
Pangamic acid (B_{15})/ dimethylglycine	Increases cardiorespiratory endurance. *Note:* This substance has been banned by the FDA; however, it is still being sold under different names.
Yohimbe	Derived from the bark of the yohimbe tree; acts as anabolic agent and aphrodisiac[†]; increases energy and strength.
Smilax	Derived from the sarsaparilla plant; acts as aphrodisiac and anabolic agent; increases athletic perfomance.

* Note that these are only claims, not research supported effects.

[†] There is some research evidence for its use in certain populations; see A Way of Life Library for further information.

Fat-Free Foods

A new weapon in the war against fat calories is the development of fat-free foods. The advertisements for these products frequently send this message: "Eat all you want because there is no fat." The problem is that overeating anything, whether it contains fat or not, will still cause you to gain weight. A calorie is a calorie regardless of whether it comes from fat. The goal of good nutrition is to not overindulge in any foods, even those that are fat-free. Variety and moderation should be the rule of thumb.

Along with the fat-free foods has come the development of fat substitutes like **olestra.** Fat substitutes are "fake" fats—they give low-fat foods the same texture and taste as their fat-ladened counterparts, but with fewer calories. The idea is to help people lose body fat. Ironically previous experience with low-calorie sweeteners does not support this theory. Following the expanded use of these sweeteners in the 1980s, obesity rates actually jumped by 30 percent! The problem is that low-calorie food additives are giving people excuses not to change their poor eating habits.

Regardless of whether fat substitutes will prove effective in the battle of the bulge, they pose another set of problems. For example, even though olestra was approved by the FDA, many nutritionists question the thoroughness with which it was tested. They claim that we simply do not know the long-term effects of eating olestra. There is already evidence that olestra can cause gastric upset and may rob the body of important compounds that help protect it from certain cancers. In fact, the labeling on foods containing olestra states "Olestra may cause abdominal cramping and loose stools. Olestra inhibits the absorption of some vitamins (A, D, E, K) and other nutrients." Why take the chance? Remember, a balanced diet is not a diet totally free of fat, but one in which 30 percent or less of the total calories comes from fat. Why be guinea pigs for substances we know little about merely because we do not want to practice restraint in our diets? Once again, moderation and variety are the keys to good nutrition.

Not Just How Much You Eat, but What You Eat

Your energy intake (food) and energy output (physical activity) must be kept in balance to keep you from gaining fat. When you eat more than you need to based on your daily energy requirements (positive energy balance), the excess energy is stored as fat; when you eat less (negative energy balance), you burn the stored fat for energy. Thus it is always important to pay attention to food portion sizes in order to achieve a negative energy balance. Too often, we are unaware of what constitutes "one serving" of a particular food. We read the nutritional information on the package, noting calories and fat, yet we frequently ignore the serving size on which these numbers are based. Quoted portion sizes are often much smaller than real-life portions. *Portion size must be monitored in all healthy diets,* particularly those geared toward body fat reduction.

Although a negative energy balance can work to reduce body fat, recent studies indicate that the composition of your diet may also be an important key to keeping off fat. Dietary fat and sugar tend to promote fatness due to hormonal influences caused by their ingestion. However, complex carbohydrates and dietary fiber, when included in the diet, tend to assist in fat loss. The point is that food intake that is low in fat and sugar appears to be a key factor in successful fat loss and healthy body composition. Therefore avoid high-fat foods and eat complex carbohydrates. For example, include such complex carbohydrates as potatoes, breads, and beans, and avoid sugary carbohydrates, such as candies, syrups, and regular soda pop. This does not mean that you have to give up grilled pork chops and cookies forever. It simply means that you need to eat less of such high-fat foods and high-sugar products (see Figure 10.1). Nutritional charts listing the fat, sugar, and caloric content of typical foods are quite useful, and many of the books listed in A Way of Life Library provide easy-to-understand tables for those who want more information.

Food, Energy, and Exercise

Now that you understand the right foods for your body, the next step is to realize that all the energy released from food eventually becomes heat. By measuring the amount of heat given off, we can determine the amount of energy released from foods or the amount of energy required for exercise. The unit of measure for energy is the **calorie** (often called a kilocalorie).

The energy needs of the body depend on factors such as body size, body composition, age, and type and amount of daily physical activity. Your **basal metabolic rate (BMR)** plus your energy needs for daily activities combine to represent your daily caloric requirement. BMR is the minimum level of energy required to sustain life at complete rest. BMR is determined usually under stringent laboratory conditions by measuring the amount of oxygen consumed during a period of complete rest at least 12 hours after the last meal.

How does the amount of oxygen consumed help us determine how many calories are required to sustain life? The oxygen consumed by your body is used to metabolize the foods we eat for energy. Therefore **oxygen consumption** can represent the amount of energy the body is expending. Most authorities set the basal oxygen requirement of the body at 3.5 milliliters per kilogram of body weight per minute. It has been established that one kilogram (2.2 pounds) of body weight burns approximately 1 calorie per hour. Knowing your weight in kilograms, you can roughly estimate your BMR. A 77-kilogram (170-pound) man, for example, would use 77 calories per hour and have a BMR of about 1,848 calories per day. To check the accuracy of this figure, we can calculate it another way since we know that 1 liter of oxygen consumed equals 4.82 calories. Using a BMR of 3.5 milliliters of oxygen per kilogram per minute, we get a total figure of 77.6 calories per hour, or 1,862 calories every 24 hours—a very close agreement.

The BMR for a woman is calculated in the same manner, only with a 10 percent reduction. Thus a 55-kilogram (121-pound) woman would utilize just under 1,200 calories a day ($0.90 \times 55 \times 24$).

WAY OF LIFE
Evaluating an Eating Plan for Body Fat Reduction

- Does the plan provide at least 1,200 calories per day?
- Does it follow Food Guide Pyramid recommendations?
- Does it claim weight loss of not more than 2 pounds per week?

- Does it recommend regular exercise as part of the program?
- Does it fit comfortably into your lifestyle?

Use your BMR to help determine how many calories to eat in order to maintain your weight. To the BMR you must add the caloric costs for the various activities performed during your day. The total represents your 24-hour caloric expenditure. Individual daily caloric expenditures (and therefore, daily caloric intake requirements) vary considerably because of differences in job requirements and recreational pursuits. Table 10.2 provides an estimate of total daily caloric expenditures for men and women of different body weights and activity levels. Note that the lighter you are or the less active you are, the fewer calories you require per day.

To estimate your caloric needs, follow the steps presented above for determining your BMR. Then, using Table 10.2, select the activity level that best describes your daily lifestyle. For instance, if you choose 60 percent, multiply your BMR for 24 hours by 0.6. Add the result to your BMR. The total is an estimate of your daily caloric expenditure. In order to maintain your present body composition, your daily caloric intake should equal the daily caloric expenditure you have calculated. If you want to lose fat, you should reduce your daily intake of calories and increase your activity level (to burn more calories). By following the exercise recommendations provided in the previous chapters and developing sensible eating habits, you either lose weight or maintain a healthy weight for a lifetime.

Energy Expenditure During Exercise

Recall that the heart rate during exercise is a direct reflection of intensity and the increased energy expenditure over that expended during rest. Accompanying the increased heart rate is an increase in **cardiac output,** which is the amount of blood pumped, and also an increase in oxygen uptake by the muscle cells being worked. The energy released during muscle contraction is known as the energy expenditure, or caloric cost, of an activity.

TABLE 10.2
Estimated Daily Caloric Expenditure Based on Body Weight and Activity Level* (calories per 24 hours)

Activity Level	Body Weight, Men				Body Weight, Women			
	60 kg (132 lb)	70 kg (154 lb)	80 kg (176 lb)	90 kg (198 lb)	50 kg (110 lb)	55 kg (121 lb)	60 kg (132 lb)	65 kg (143 lb)
40% *Sedentary:* sitting most of the day; limited walking	2,030	2,370	2,710	3,050	1,520	1,680	1,830	1,980
50% *Semisedentary:* sitting, standing, walking, and limited other physical activities	2,180	2,540	2,900	3,270	1,630	1,790	1,960	2,120
60% *Light to moderate:* everyday class and work activities; sporadic or weekend sports and physical activities	2,320	2,710	3,100	3,480	1,740	1,910	2,090	2,260
70% *Moderate to vigorous:* regular participation in fitness exercise, intramural sports, or other physical activities	2,470	2,880	3,290	3,700	1,850	2,030	2,220	2,400
80% *Very active:* regular vigorous cardiorespiratory physical activity, four or more times a week, at 70 percent HR reserve, for 30 minutes or more	2,610	3,050	3,480	3,920	1,960	2,150	2,350	2,550

* Calculations are based on a basal oxygen requirement of 3.5 milliliters of oxygen for each kilogram of body weight per minute and on a caloric equivalent of 4.8 calories per liter of oxygen used. (Values listed have been rounded off to the nearest 10 calories.)

Caloric cost can be calculated if we measure the amount of heat given off by the body. However, during exercise, this task has proven to be extremely difficult. During the late nineteenth century, a scientist related the heat loss from energy expenditure to the amount of oxygen consumed by the body. From this research, a method called **indirect calorimetry** has been devised for measuring energy expenditure. Using it, we can calculate the number of calories expended by determining the amount of oxygen utilized.

In recent years, much research has been devoted to establishing the energy costs of various sports and fitness activities. When estimating energy expenditure for any individual, we must consider the time spent doing the activity, the intensity, body size, and the amount of muscle mass involved. The more time you spend at an activity, the more energy you use. Higher intensities require more energy than lesser intensities. Larger people tend to require more energy than smaller people for the same task. And activities involving a large amount of muscle mass burn more calories than those involving limited muscle mass.

Energy Cost of Running

Table 10.3 presents values for specific running speeds in cal/min./kg as well as in cal/min. for 120-, 150-, and 180-pound persons. To estimate your energy cost for running, first determine your kilogram body weight by multiplying your weight in pounds by 0.45 (1 pound equals 0.45 kilograms). Next, select your preferred running speed. Multiply your kilogram weight by the value under the column headed "Cal/min./kg" in Table 10.3. This will give your per-minute caloric cost.

In addition, each running speed is expressed in terms of METS, another measure of intensity. METS differ from calories by providing the additional information of how an activity's energy expenditure compares to that at rest. One **MET** is equivalent to the energy needed at rest, or approximately 1.25 calories (about a quarter of a liter of oxygen) per minute. Classifying an activity at 7 METS, for instance, means that it requires seven times more energy than sitting in a chair at rest. Seven METS would be at the high end of moderate exercise; it is equivalent to 8.8 calories per minute, or a little more than 1.75 liters of oxygen uptake. Anything over 9 METS is considered vigorous activity. Marathon runners, who probably represent the zenith of cardiorespiratory fitness, run for 2 to 3 hours at an intensity level of 12 to 15 METS or more.

Other factors affect caloric expenditure. For example, a 170-pound man (76.5 kg) running at a 10-minute-per-mile pace would require 11.3 calories per minute. This is a greater caloric cost than for a woman running at the same pace. The reason for the higher cost is that the man is carrying more total body mass (and probably more muscle mass) and thus requires more energy. Nevertheless, the man's heart-rate response to this activity may or may not be in his target heart-rate range; it all depends on his physical fitness. The better

TABLE 10.3 Energy Cost of Running					
		Cal/min.			
Speed	**Cal/min./kg**	**120-lb Person (54 kg)**	**150-lb Person (68 kg)**	**180-lb Person (81 kg)**	**METS**
10-min. mile (6 mph)	0.1471	7.9	10.0	11.9	6–10
8-min. mile (7.5 mph)	0.1856	10.0	12.6	15.0	8–12
7-min. mile (8.6 mph)	0.2118	11.4	14.4	17.2	9–14
6-min. mile (10 mph)	0.2350	12.7	16.0	19.0	10–15

conditioned you are, the greater the caloric expenditure you can muster in a given period of time. For example, contrast two men, both weighing 68 kilograms. One can run 4 miles in 28 minutes (a 7-minute-per-mile pace) at a heart rate of 150 (an adequate training stimulus). The other can only run 2.8 miles during the same time period (28 minutes at a 10-minute-per-mile pace) and at the same heart rate of 150. The first runner utilizes 493 calories for his workout; the second man can utilize only 280 calories during his workout. We can readily see that the man in better physical condition burns more calories during his workout than the slower runner does.

Now assume that the slower runner runs 4 miles, or the same total distance as the 7-minute miler. He would then use another 120 calories, which would give him a similar caloric expenditure of 400 calories. However, his total workout time is 49 minutes rather than 28. Obviously the runner who can run the 4 miles in 28 minutes has a greater functional fitness capacity than the slower man. Nevertheless, when burning calories with running, the distance you move is more important than your speed.

Energy Cost of Selected Physical Activities

Table 10.4 gives energy costs for a variety of physical activities expressed in calories per minute for a 150-pound person and in calories per minute per kilogram of body weight. You can use Table 10.4 to estimate your energy cost for any of the activities listed. Simply refer to the values in the "Cal/min./kg" column, multiplying your body weight in kilograms to get a per-minute caloric value. Activities are listed in ascending order from less intense (such as archery) to the most intense (running a 6-minute mile). Activities that require

TABLE 10.4
Energy Costs for Selected Physical Activities (for a 150-pound person)

Activity	Cal/min./kg	Cal/min.	METS
Archery (American Round)	0.0412	2.8	2.3
Bowling (with three other bowlers)	0.0471	3.2	2.7
Golf (playing in a foursome)	0.0559	3.8	3.2
Walking (17-min. mile on a grass surface)	0.0794	5.4	4.5
Stepping (8-inch bench)	0.0823	5.6	4.7
Cycling (6.4-min. mile)	0.0985	6.7	5.6
Canoeing (15-min. mile)	0.1029	7.0	5.8
Aerobics (moderate)	0.103	7.0	5.8
In-line skating (10 mph)	0.1294	8.8	7.4
Swimming (50-yd/min.)	0.1333	9.1	7.6
Running (10-min. mile)	0.1471	10.0	8.0
Cycling (5-min. mile)	0.1559	10.6	8.5
Handball (singles)	0.1603	10.9	9.1
Skipping rope (80 turns/min.)	0.1655	11.3	9.5
Rowing (28–32 strokes/min.)	0.1856	12.6	10.0
Running (8-min. mile)	0.1856	12.6	10.0
Cross-country skiing (intense)	0.200	13.6	12.0
Running (6-min. mile)	0.2350	16.0	12.8

Source: Based on personal research and, in some cases, on research reported
in professional journals.

5 to 9 calories per minute (1.0 to 1.8 liters of oxygen) are classified as moderate. Activities requiring above 9 calories per minute are classified as vigorous.

Activities of below-moderate intensity, such as golf and archery, do not represent a suitable means for developing or maintaining physical fitness. In these activities, the stress on the cardiorespiratory and muscular systems is not great enough to produce a training effect. For burning calories, however, activities such as golf can be beneficial. Although the cardiac and respiratory stimulus is minimal, you do burn more calories than if you engaged in a sedentary activity like watching television. However, if we compare the 68-kilogram runner who runs 4 miles in 28 minutes (a caloric cost of 493 calories) with a golfer of the same weight, we find that the golfer must play for a total of 106 minutes to burn the same 493 calories. Put another way, the golfer has to exercise nearly four times as long for the same energy cost benefits.

Guidelines for Healthy Body Composition

When it comes to food, we all need the same nutrients, but in different amounts. Young people need greater quantities of food for body growth and upkeep and for energy. Men generally need more food than women, due in part to their larger percentage of lean body mass. Large people need more food than small people. However, when people overeat—that is, when they take in more calories than their daily activities use up—they gain fat. As discussed previously, intake of food in excess of our daily needs leads to overfatness. Nearly half of all American adults are overfat, with studies indicating that the number is increasing.

Obesity is an extreme level of overfatness and is a major public health problem. Obesity is clinically defined as having 25 percent or more body fat for men and 30 percent or more body fat for women. As the most prevalent form of malnutrition in the United States, obesity has far-reaching complications. It is closely related to cardiovascular, respiratory, kidney, and gall bladder diseases, as well as to diabetes, disorders of the bones and joints, and, for some people, emotional imbalance. It also increases the risk for complications during surgery. Obese persons are more prone to fatigue (increasing the risk of accidents), indigestion, and constipation, and they have disproportionate numbers of aches and pains. Besides having to cope with the psychological effects of being fat, they face premature death.

Many people like to believe that some metabolic abnormality is the reason for their being obese. Most often, this is not true. Medical research does not support the popular notion that endocrine malfunction is the reason for obesity. Instead, evidence is accumulating that a sedentary lifestyle is the real culprit. The obese simply do not burn off the calories they consume each day, and this surplus energy is stored as fat deposits in the body.

A consideration for those of you who are parents or about to be is the danger of allowing your children to become fat at an early age. Recent research indicates that human fat cells increase in number very rapidly in early life and, once formed, become fixed for life. Pediatricians are increasingly concerned over this fact. Overfeeding tends to rapidly multiply the number of fat cells in young children, making it more difficult for them to control body fat throughout life. To curb this potential for fatness, proper eating and exercise habits should be cultivated at an early age. *Managing body fat is a lifetime affair, beginning with a parent's concern, instruction, and perhaps most importantly, role-modeling.*

In determining a desirable and healthy weight, it is more important to know how fat you are rather than how much you weigh. The standard age-height-weight tables are derived from measurements of a great number of people.

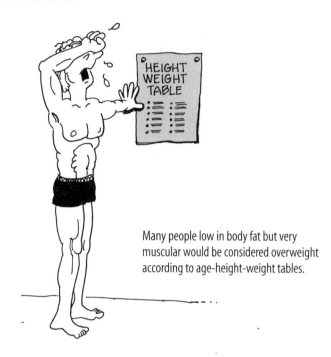

Many people low in body fat but very muscular would be considered overweight according to age-height-weight tables.

Although these charts enable each person to make comparisons with the average man or woman, they are often inadequate guides for figuring a healthy weight. Many athletes, low in body fat but very muscular, would be overweight according to these charts. Also, most of these age-height-weight charts allow small increases in body weight with increasing age, a practice that lacks scientific justification.

Without question, it is the proportion of fat tissue in your body, and not your scale weight, that determines your proper weight. Methods have been developed for measuring the relative leanness or fatness of the body. Values for body composition obtained from such laboratory assessments as skinfold measurements and underwater weighing can be used to classify your relative fatness. Once you measure your body fat, you can refer to Table 10.5, which lists body fat norms.

The Role of Exercise in Managing Body Composition

We all want to look good and feel good. Studies on managing body composition point to the overwhelming success of combining sensible eating with regular exercise rather than relying solely on one component. While reducing the

TABLE 10.5 Norms for Body Composition		
Classification	Women (% body fat)	Men (% body fat)
Desirable	16 – 25	12 – 20
Overfat	25.1 – 34.9	20.1 – 24.9
Obese	≥35	≥25

amount of food you eat may help you lose weight, physical activity is necessary to maintain your ideal body composition. Exercise is the key to increasing your muscle mass, to burning enough calories so that you don't have to starve yourself, and to stoking your metabolism to a higher degree.

The importance of regular exercise in managing the amount of body fat and lean mass we each possess is well accepted today. Physical activity is the great variable in energy expenditure and can play a key role in controlling your body fat. To try to maintain a desirable body composition while living a sedentary life would probably mean lifelong hunger and a flabby, poorly toned body.

A significant amount of the weight, as measured on a scale, that is lost from dieting alone comes from body water and lean (not fat) body tissue. Many people on a low-carbohydrate diet, which depletes stored carbohydrates, experience quick weight loss due to an associated loss of body water. They are encouraged by what they see on the scale, but in fact they are being deceived. Such crash diets often result in the loss of lean body tissue from muscles, bones, and organs. When the crash diet ends and normal eating resumes, weight is regained, mostly as fat (it takes longer to rebuild lean body tissues). And when the weight is regained, the dieting often begins again. People who constantly undergo these "yo-yo diets" can become so frustrated that they simply give up.

When you start an exercise program, you can expect slight gains in muscle tissue. Even when you lose body fat, your total body weight may not change as quickly as you would expect due to this increase in lean body mass. This disappoints some people because they do not see the needle drop on their bathroom scales as much as they would expect. However, you may see a loss of inches in your girths and increased muscle tone, and your clothes may fit looser. So don't be discouraged. The right kind of weight loss is occurring. Realize that the burning off of stored fat continues if your energy expenditures exceed the amount of calories you consume. To confirm your positive change in body composition, perhaps you should be reassessed with a laboratory technique such as a skinfold test or an underwater weighing procedure.

Studies have demonstrated that today's adults are increasingly less active than their counterparts in years gone by. Many people experience "creeping obesity," the gradual yet significant increase in fat over a period of years that is caused mainly by inactivity. Studies comparing obese with nonobese subjects have demonstrated that *the cause of fatness is usually an inactive lifestyle, not increased food consumption.* In fact, people who are active and lean tend to eat more than inactive and obese persons. The fat content of a fit individual's meals also tends to be less than that of an obese individual.

Misconceptions About Exercise and Fat Loss

Despite research evidence, several misconceptions about the relationship between exercise and fat loss still exist. Following is a brief discussion of a few of the more commonly held misconceptions.

Exercise and Appetite

Often we hear that if you exercise more, you will eat more. Research studies have concluded that regular fitness-related exercise sessions do not bring about a corresponding increase in appetite and food intake. Appetite, the psychological desire for food, often is triggered even when you are not hungry. Therefore it does not follow that if you are inactive, you will eat less than if you were active. Research suggests that sedentary people tend to take in more food (energy) than they use, with fatness resulting. In people with a normal range of activity, appetite and exercise are attuned to each other. Some individuals even find that vigorous exercise actually suppresses their appetites for a period of time following a workout and so schedule exercise sessions to precede meals that tend to be troublesome.

Spot Reducing

Health spas and weight reduction salons of the past often promoted spot-reducing programs. Women, especially, were encouraged to use localized exercise or mechanical gadgets to reduce the fatty stores in the areas of greater fat deposition. If such spot reductions were possible, people with chubby faces could simply chew gum to "exercise" their way to lean profiles! Fortunately today's consumers are more aware that the claims made for such programs and devices are spurious. To date, the research does not support the theory that if you exercise a particular area of your body, you will reduce the excess fat in that region. Calisthenics (using body weight as resistance), yoga, and "body sculpting," although beneficial in developing general muscular endurance and strength and flexibility, do not spot reduce.

Several studies have indicated that regular vigorous and continuous exercise that involves total body movement does reduce skinfold fat and girth mea-

WAY OF LIFE
Wishful Thinking

- Dehydration is useless for controlling body fat and can be dangerous.

surements. The loss of fat, however, tends to be from all over the body. Resistance training for increased muscle tone combined with activities that vigorously stress the cardiorespiratory system provide the best means for reducing fat and achieving a lean body. Do not forget, however, that any exercise program developed to reduce body fat must be accompanied by reduced caloric intake. It is very difficult to use up enough energy by exercising to offset out-of-control eating.

Fat Reduction by Sweating

Many people purposely overheat their bodies, hoping for a quick loss of excess body fat. Exercising in hot, humid weather, or exercising while wearing a rubber or nylon sweat suit, or even sitting in a steam room after exercise are common methods for prompting profuse sweating. Although the reading on the scales may be temporarily lower by a pound or two, this weight loss has nothing to do with body fat and will not be permanent. Basically heavy sweating accomplishes only one thing: a greater-than-normal loss of water from the body. This water loss, especially if excessive, can become life-threatening. Why? A rubber suit, or any unneeded extra clothing, does not allow the heat produced during exercise to escape from the body. Likewise a steam room or a hot, humid environment diminishes the body's capacity to dispel heat normally. It is important to understand that evaporation of sweat is the major means of heat dissipation during vigorous exercise. When you wear a rubber suit, the sweat does not evaporate, causing your body temperature to become higher than normal. When the heat produced by the exercising muscles cannot be eliminated properly, the body's heat-regulating mechanisms are overburdened. This leads to a loss of too much body water, a decrease in blood volume, a severe rise in body temperature, and possible circulatory collapse.

The key point here is that dehydration (removal of body water) is useless for fat control and can be dangerous. If you purposely dehydrate, you will restore the depleted body water in a few hours when you eat and drink. Water does not contain calories, and excess body fat is lost only by burning calories, not by losing water. Tampering with the heat balance of the body can be risky. But sweating itself is not a hazard; it is a necessary mechanism for maintaining heat balance during physical activity.

Combining Exercise and Decreased Caloric Intake

Using exercise or diet alone to reduce body fat can prove to be difficult and time-consuming. *To lose 1 pound of fat, you must expend 3,500 calories more than you consume.* This would be the equivalent caloric expenditure of running about 35 miles! If your goal is to lose 1 pound per week using exercise alone, you would have to burn 500 calories more than usual every day that week (7 × 500). Even if you exercised vigorously for 30 minutes, you would be hard-pressed to burn 500 calories and would have to extend your duration to 45 to 60 minutes. Or, if you chose not to exercise and used decreased caloric intake alone, not only would you have to decrease your daily caloric intake by 500 calories, you would also risk losing some lean body mass. However, when you combine exercise and decreased caloric intake, you can maintain or even increase your lean body mass.

Therefore take a long-range view of your situation. Exercise daily at a more reasonable caloric expenditure level of 300 calories (one you can endure), and reduce your caloric intake by 200 calories, and that 1 pound of fat loss is much more easily attained and maintained. Another method is to exercise four days per week at 450 calories per session and also reduce your daily food intake by 450 calories for a 3,600 calorie deficit per week. *Losing 1 to 2 pounds of body fat per week is a reasonable goal for most individuals.* If more weight is lost, it is questionable whether it is entirely fat weight. For those anxious to lose fat, this recommendation may seem too slow. However, experience has demonstrated that if you lose body fat gradually and systematically, you are more likely to keep it off. It allows you to modify your eating habits and activity levels in sensible increments—as choices you can live with now and in the future.

Determining Your Ideal Body Weight

Once you determine your current body-fat level and decide what level you would like to achieve, there is nothing wrong with having a body weight goal as long as you lose fat as recommended here. Due to daily scale weight fluctuations, weigh yourself only once a week at the same time of day and using the same scale each time. When you reach your goal, reassess your percentage of body fat with the same accurate measuring technique you used initially (skinfolds or underwater weighing). To determine your ideal body weight based on your desired level of body fat, a simple calculation can be performed:

1. Multiply your current weight by your percentage of body fat to determine your fat weight.
2. Subtract your fat weight from your total weight to determine your lean body weight.
3. Divide your lean weight by 1 minus your desired percentage of body fat to determine your ideal body weight.

Let's take an example. Suppose a young man weighs 189 pounds, and his percentage of body fat is estimated at 23 percent. This works out to 43 pounds of body fat (0.23 × 189) and 146 pounds of lean body weight (189 − 43). To calculate his ideal body weight at his desired goal of 12 percent body fat, we simply divide the lean body weight by 0.88 (1 − 0.12). We get a value of 165 pounds as his desired body weight. If this man follows the recommendation of losing 1 to 2 pounds of body fat per week, he can plan on reaching his desired percentage of body fat in 12 to 24 weeks.

Summary

Food has always been a focal point of our lives. Although a necessity, eating has also been viewed as a recreational activity, something we do in leisure time for pleasure. We snack in front of the TV set or as we study. We go out to eat at our favorite pizza parlors and fast-food restaurants. Preparation of hearty meals is a way of showing affection for others; holiday feasts and backyard barbecues are affairs we look forward to. Business transactions are frequently conducted over meals. The result of all this enjoyable eating can be excess fat or even outright obesity.

We live in a society that has become increasingly inactive as technology has advanced. Today sedentary living is encouraged by the continued development of work-saving equipment and passive amusements and recreations. But the body was made to be active, and it thrives on movement and vigorous activity. An active lifestyle should be programmed into your daily living plan to counter the effects of technological advances and inactive recreational pursuits. You need to blend proper eating habits with vigorous exercise to develop and maintain a healthy functioning body.

Obesity and inactivity have been correlated with coronary heart disease, high blood pressure, diabetes, and other degenerative disorders. But obesity and overfatness are virtually unknown among vigorous, active people. Athletes, fitness enthusiasts, and active sportspeople seldom have excess body fat. Almost everyone is concerned about their body fat and their appearance, and many people go on diets when they become overfat. However, research has shown convincingly that diets do not work. Rather, eating better and exercising more, combined with an overall commitment to living better, do work. The goal is not merely to lose fat, but to keep it off, or better still, to never put it on. Now is the time to establish sound nutritional and exercise habits. Don't wait until your health and fitness have deteriorated.

Your daily food fare should contain low levels of fat, with special attention to restricting saturated fats and cholesterol. Increase your levels of complex carbohydrates. Avoid foods high in sugar. Eat moderate amounts of protein. Find a balance between physical activity and your caloric intake to help maintain an appropriate body composition for you.

Key Words

AMINO ACIDS: The basic building blocks of protein.

BASAL METABOLIC RATE (BMR): The minimal level of energy required to sustain life at complete rest.

BLOOD SUGAR: The glucose found in the blood which is used for energy or stored as glycogen in cells.

CALORIE: A unit of measure for the rate of heat or energy production in the body from food; often called a kilocalorie.

CARBOHYDRATES: A food substance that is the primary energy food for vigorous muscular activity; includes various sugars and starches and is found in the body in the form of glucose and glycogen.

CARDIAC OUTPUT: The amount of blood pumped in 1 minute by the heart.

ENERGY EXPENDITURE: The energy released during exercise; often referred to as caloric cost.

FAT: A food substance that is a source of energy in the body; an insulator and protector of vital organs.

FATTY ACID: The end product of the breakdown of fats in the body.

GLUCOSE: A type of carbohydrate that is transported in the blood and metabolized in the cell; also called blood sugar.

GLYCOGEN: The storage form of carbohydrates found in the liver and muscles.

INDIRECT CALORIMETRY: A method for measuring energy expenditure by relating the heat loss from energy expenditure to the amount of oxygen consumed by the body; it can be used to calculate the number of calories expended during a given activity by determining the amount of oxygen utilized; 1 liter of oxygen = 4.82 calories.

MET: The rate of energy expended at rest in 1 minute; used to rate activities in multiples above the resting rate; 3.5 milliliters of oxygen per kilogram body weight per minute.

MINERALS: A group of 22 metallic elements vital to proper cell functioning.

NUTRIENTS: The basic substances needed by the body that are provided by eating food.

NUTRITION: The foods we eat and how our bodies process them.

NUTRITIONAL ERGOGENIC AIDS: Special foods or supplements that are touted to improve physical fitness levels or athletic performance.

OBESITY: The state of being too fat; males $\geq 25\%$ and females $\geq 35\%$ fat.

OLESTRA: A fat substitute; "fake fat."

OXYGEN UPTAKE: The consumption of oxygen, indicating the amount of energy the body uses; 1 liter of oxygen = 4.8 calories.

PROTEIN: A food substance that provides the basic structural components of cells and is also the source for enzymes and hormones in the body.

SATURATED FATS: A food source found in meat, whole milk, cheese, and butter; are solid at room temperature.

TRIGLYCERIDES: The most common form of fat found in the body; composed of three fatty acids.

UNSATURATED FATS: A liquid type of fat found in peanut oil and olive oil.

VITAMINS: Organic substances that perform vital functions within the cells.

A Way of Life Library

Anderson, J., and B. Deskins. *The Nutrition Bible.* New York: Morrow, 1995.

Bellerson, K. J. *The Complete and Up-to-Date Fat Book.* Garden City Park, NY: Avery, 1993.

Bucci, L. R., Ed. *Nutrients as Ergogenic Aids for Sports and Exercise.* Boca Raton, FL: CRC Press, 1993.

Center for Science in the Public Interest. *Nutrition Action Newsletter.* Washington, DC: CSPI. (1-800-237–4874.)

Clark, N. *Nancy Clark's Sports Nutrition Guidebook.* Champaign, IL: Human Kinetics, 1990.

Cooper, K. H. *Antioxidant Revolution.* Nashville, TN: Nelson, 1994.

Katch, F. I., and W. D. McArdle. *Nutrition, Weight Control, and Exercise.* 4th ed. Philadelphia: Lea & Febiger, 1992.

Kostas, G. G. *The Balancing Act Nutrition and Weight Guide.* Dallas: Arcata Graphics,1993.

Netzer, C. T. *The Complete Book of Food Counts.* New York: Dell, 1988.

Pennington, J. A. T. *Bowes and Church's Food Values of Portions Commonly Used,* 15th ed. New York: HarperCollins, 1989.

Tribole, E. *Eating on the Run,* 2nd ed. Champaign, IL: Human Kinetics, 1992.

Wolinsky, I., and J. F. Hickson, Jr., eds. *Nutrition in Exercise and Sport,* 2nd ed. Boca Raton, FL: CRC Press, 1994.

CHAPTER *11*

Exercise and Heart Disease

Although there has been a decline in recent years in the heart disease mortality rate among Americans, heart disease is still the single leading killer. Equally distressing is the fact that approximately 45 percent of all heart attack victims are under age 65, and 5 percent are under age 40. In the past, the death rates for men were always higher than those for women. However, over the last decade, the death rate from heart attack

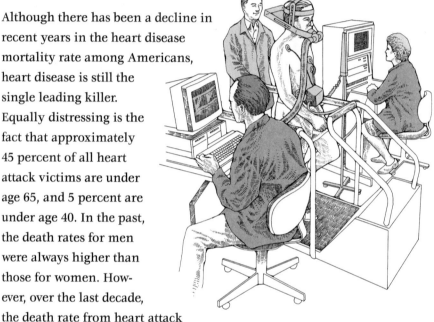

for women has increased to nearly 49 percent of all cases, almost equal to that of men.

As you read this chapter, keep these statements in mind:

- Heart disease occurs when the coronary arteries (the blood vessels that supply the heart muscle with nutrients and oxygen) are impaired by a buildup of cholesterol and associated fatty substances on the inner portion of the artery wall. Such accumulations, often referred to as atherosclerosis, tend to limit the blood flow to the heart muscle and, if severe enough, can lead to heart attack.

- Medical research has identified certain risk factors associated with an increased incidence of atherosclerosis. High blood pressure, smoking, a high level of fats in the blood (cholesterol), and lack of exercise (inactivity) are the major risk factors for the development of coronary heart disease.

- Many other variables such as obesity, diabetes, everyday tensions, and a diet high in saturated fats have also been correlated with atherosclerosis.
- One's age, sex, race, and heredity are risk factors that cannot be controlled or remedied. However, proper diet and exercise offer some protection against the early appearance of heart disease.
- Vigorous regular exercise appears to have much potential for adding more life to your years and possibly more years to your life.

Coronary heart disease is the leading cause of death in the United States today. Recently the American Heart Association estimated that as many as 1.5 million Americans have heart attacks each year, resulting in more than 500,000 deaths. The American mortality rate from heart disease is one of the highest in the world. According to estimates by the American Heart Association, one in four Americans have one or more forms of cardiovascular disease. Despite significant advances in the diagnosis and treatment of heart disease, the unfortunate fact is that the number of deaths from heart disease has declined only slightly in recent years. Equally discouraging is the fact that 45 percent of all heart attacks occur in people under age 65. The mortality rates for men have always been higher than those for women. However, the number of deaths from heart disease among American women has increased greatly in recent years.

Some experts call heart disease the "disease of prosperity"; others label it the "abuse of our prosperity." Technological and scientific advances certainly have raised our living standard. However, the resultant soft living has made us vulnerable to heart disease. Research is showing that regular exercise along with prudent dietary modifications can help reduce the risk of heart disease.

Atherosclerosis

The heart is a sturdy, tough muscle; it contracts 100,000 times a day with enough force to pump blood through 60,000 miles of blood vessels. But the blood pumped through the heart does not nourish the heart itself. Instead the heart muscle is supplied with blood through its own system, the coronary arteries. **Coronary heart disease** occurs when these arteries are impaired by a buildup of **cholesterol** and associated fatty substances on the inner portion of the artery walls. These deposits cause a thickening of the inner walls and a serious narrowing of the blood vessels, a condition called **atherosclerosis.** In later stages, these deposits cause the arteries to lose their pliability, which leads to a hardening of the vessels, a condition called **arteriosclerosis.** When such accumulations occur in the coronary arteries, they limit the blood flow to the heart muscle (see Figure 11.1). When the blockage becomes severe, the heart can suffer a **myocardial infarction** (heart attack), which results in the death

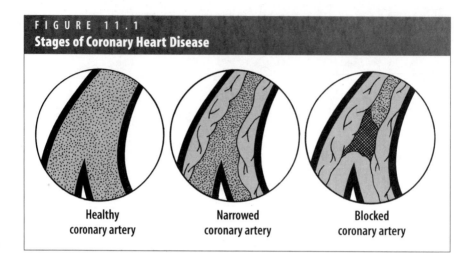

FIGURE 11.1
Stages of Coronary Heart Disease

| Healthy coronary artery | Narrowed coronary artery | Blocked coronary artery |

of part of the heart muscle. This malfunction may seem sudden, but it has actually been building up for years.

The best evidence of the early and gradual accumulation of fatty deposits in the body's arteries is a much-quoted autopsy study of U.S. soldiers killed in the Korean War. The subjects averaged only 22 years of age, but 77 percent of them showed signs of disease of the coronary arteries, varying from a slight thickening of the artery linings to complete occlusion (blockage) of one or more main artery branches. A substantial proportion of these young Americans had impaired circulation long before any symptoms would have appeared. Interestingly comparable studies of Korean soldiers killed alongside the Americans revealed no evidence of similar coronary damage. Studies in other countries (such as autopsies of accident victims) have also shown that early arteriosclerosis is more common in young American men than it is elsewhere in the world. Data on combat casualties in Vietnam indicated significant cardiovascular disease in nearly 50 percent of the victims.

Based on this evidence, we must recognize that coronary heart disease is not simply a disease of the elderly. Instead this deadly buildup of fatty substances in the arteries begins at an early age. Some pediatricians believe that preventive measures should begin in childhood and perhaps even in infancy. Heart disease doesn't just happen overnight; more and more evidence now suggests that it begins in childhood and can lead to a heart attack in the prime of life.

Statistics over the past decade indicate a decline in the death rates from diseases of the heart and circulation. Credit for this must be given to advances in research, professional care, public education, and the development of community programs sponsored by the American Heart Association and other agencies. Such programs are aimed at improving the knowledge of and services for dealing with these life-threatening diseases of the heart and blood vessels. The AHA has recently taken a strong stance on the benefits of regular exercise for the health of your heart and circulation.

According to the AHA, the latest scientific evidence confirms that regular aerobic (cardiorespiratory) exercise plays a significant role in decreasing the risk for heart and blood vessel disease. Thus *inactivity is now cited as one of the four major risk factors for heart disease,* the others being high blood pressure, smoking, and high cholesterol levels. However, much more still needs to be done to help people modify their lifestyles in a healthful way.

Coronary Risk Factors

The term **risk** refers to the possibility or chance that something bad will happen. In the area of health, risk is often expressed in degrees of danger. Scientists use statistics to determine the possibility, or odds, that something will occur. Information about the possibility of having a health problem is called a statistical risk. A statistical risk is based on what has happened to a group of people in the recent past. From such data, you can evaluate your degree of risk for, in this case, early heart disease. Risk factors associated with an increased incidence of atherosclerosis have been identified. The greater the number of these coronary risk factors one has, the greater one's chance for heart disease, and perhaps premature death. **Hypertension** (high blood pressure), high levels of cholesterol and triglycerides in the blood, cigarette smoking, a high intake of saturated fats, obesity, emotional problems, and physical inactivity have all been linked to coronary heart disease. Other factors include one's age, sex, race, and heredity. The latter are predetermined and cannot be controlled or remedied. However, we can do something about diet, body fatness, smoking, and exercise.

Age, Sex, Race, and Heredity

The incidence of atherosclerosis and coronary heart disease increases with age. The American Heart Association estimates that one-fifth of all persons killed by cardiovascular diseases are under age 65. At ages 35 to 44, the death rate for white males from coronary heart disease is much higher than that for women. However, after menopause, the incidence of the disease for women begins to approach the level for men of comparable age. Women's diminished hormonal production after menopause is believed to account for this increased coronary disease rate.

African Americans have a higher death rate from coronary disease than white Americans do. Surprisingly African American women are stricken at an earlier age than white men or women, and even earlier than African American men. The reason for this is currently unknown.

A hereditary element is linked with coronary disease. Heart attacks, especially those that strike at an early age, appear to run in families. However, the specific genetic defects remain unknown. Some of this relationship is probably somewhat associated with one's environment. For example, fat parents usually have fat children, tense parents often have tense children, and poor dietary habits and inactive lifestyles are often family-influenced. The exact nature of the role of heredity in coronary heart disease is very complex, especially when we consider the other conditions that frequently precede coronary heart disease, such as diabetes, hypertension, and elevated serum cholesterol. In some instances, these factors can be inherited; however, they are also outcomes of one's lifestyle.

Hypertension

If you have ever had a physical examination, most likely your blood pressure has been checked. An inflatable cuff is wrapped around your upper arm, and air is pumped into the cuff. Indirectly this procedure measures the amount of pressure maintained in your arteries. The pumping ability of your heart and the resilience of your arteries influence this measurement. The pressure is recorded as two numbers. The higher number, called **systolic pressure,** is your blood pressure at the moment blood is ejected from the heart. The lower number, the **diastolic pressure,** is your blood pressure between beats when the heart is relaxed and resting. Under relaxed conditions, the pressure rises from a diastolic level of 80 mmHg (millimeters of mercury) to a systolic level of 120 mmHg. Blood pressure is capable of going up and down within a limited range (as during exercise), but when it starts high and stays high during rest, then hypertension, or high blood pressure, is present. High blood pressure, which usually means any pressures at or above 140/90, is largely unexplained. We do know that an elevated blood pressure means the heart must work harder than normal, putting an abnormal strain on the heart and arteries. This elevated pressure has been linked to heart disease, strokes, and atherosclerosis. The heart, brain, and kidneys are particularly susceptible to damage from high blood pressure. Recently developed drugs have proved effective in controlling hypertension. However, physicians are now recommending exercise and weight loss as the first steps in controlling blood pressure. Exercise has shown promising results in reducing arterial pressure.

According to American Heart Association statistics, high blood pressure causes over 35,000 deaths per year. A national health and nutrition survey estimated that as many as 50 million adults and children have high blood pressure. Unfortunately more than half of these Americans who are hypertensive do not

> **WAY OF LIFE**
> **Hypertension: The Silent Killer**
>
> - One out of every four Americans has high blood pressure.
> - Over half of those with hypertension do not know they have it.
> - Many people neglect to have their blood pressure checked regularly.
> - Early detection and treatment of high blood pressure can save lives.

know it. And many who are aware of it are not getting suitable treatment. According to the AHA, high blood pressure is nearly 50 percent more prevalent among African Americans than white Americans. African Americans, Puerto Ricans, Cuban Americans, and Mexican Americans are more likely to suffer from hypertensive heart disease than white Americans. Hypertension greatly increases the risk for suffering a heart attack or stroke. In fact, a person with a systolic blood pressure of over 150 mmHg has more than twice the risk of heart attack than a person with a systolic blood pressure under 120. *Do you know what your blood pressure is?*

Smoking

Without question, cigarette smoking is harmful to your health. In fact, *any* use of tobacco is harmful to your health and well-being. Although the number of smokers has declined more than 37 percent since 1965, over 400,000 Americans die each year from smoking-related illnesses. Tobacco use is closely linked to pulmonary emphysema, lung cancer, mouth cancer, and heart attacks. The American Heart Association states that a person who smokes more than one pack a day has nearly twice the risk of heart attack as the nonsmoker. Although the exact role that smoking plays in the development of heart attacks has not been established, cigarette smoking clearly increases the risk. Fortunately the death rate from cardiovascular disease among smokers who stop smoking is nearly as low as that of people who have never smoked.

The Centers for Disease Control and Prevention estimate that 75 percent of adult smokers started before age 18 and 90 percent began before they were 21. More recently, a survey revealed that if you have not taken up smoking prior to reaching your early twenties, the chances of your becoming a smoker are almost nil. If you are currently a smoker or are constantly exposed to second-hand smoke, you are at an increased risk for early heart disease. For the young adult, the choice to smoke or not to smoke has a major bearing on achieving a healthy lifestyle.

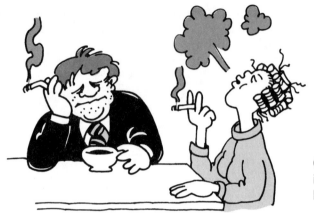

Cigarette smoking increases the risk of heart attack.

For a moment, let's disregard the health risks of tobacco use. People who smoke have smelly tobacco breath, their hair and clothes stink, their car stinks, their house stinks, and 75 percent of the population does not want to be around a smoker "in action." Perhaps this is reason enough for smokers to eliminate this unhealthy practice from their lives.

Cholesterol

The relationship between high blood cholesterol levels and heart disease has provoked much controversy in recent decades. Cholesterol is produced in the liver; it is essential for cell structure and for the formation of various hormones, including the sex hormones. However, cholesterol and other fatty substances called triglycerides also make up the atherosclerotic deposits on the inner lining of the arteries. Medical researchers believe that cholesterol floating in the blood is the source of the continual accumulation. A diet high in saturated fat increases cholesterol concentrations in the blood.

The level of total cholesterol in the blood can be measured. Elevated levels of cholesterol above 200 mg/dl (milligrams per deciliter) are associated with an increased risk for developing atherosclerosis. The National Cholesterol Education Program (NCEP) has established a total blood cholesterol value below 200 as desirable. A level of 200 to 240 is borderline to high risk, while values over 240 are high-risk and dangerous. A person with a value above 240 has about three times the risk of heart attack or stroke as a person with a cholesterol level below 200. Over 50 percent of Americans are estimated to have cholesterol values of 200 mg/dl or higher. In addition, close to 20 percent of Americans have values of 240 or above.

WAY OF LIFE
Ways to Lower Your Cholesterol Level

- Decrease total fat in your diet.
- Decrease saturated fat in your diet.
- Decrease cholesterol in your diet.

- Maintain your ideal body weight.
- Participate in regular aerobic exercise.

Diets high in animal fat and high-cholesterol foods and sedentary lifestyles are factors that correlate highly with elevated cholesterol levels. Recent evidence has demonstrated the value of replacing some of the saturated fats in the diet with polyunsaturated fats derived from vegetable sources, such as safflower oil. This adjustment in diet has tended to lower cholesterol values in some people. There is also evidence of reductions in cholesterol levels as the result of physical fitness programs. Exercise is now widely accepted as a good intervention for preventing diseases associated with elevated levels of cholesterol.

Although it is important to keep your level of cholesterol down (below 200 mg/dl), findings from several heart disease studies suggest that a more involved analysis of blood **lipids** (fats) is necessary. It may be more important to know how cholesterol is carried in the bloodstream than simply to know the total amount present. Cholesterol is carried in the bloodstream by certain proteins. Because these proteins are carrying lipids, they are called **lipoproteins.** Two types of lipoprotein are especially important in heart disease: **high-density lipoprotein (IIDL)** and **low-density lipoprotein (LDL).** The LDLs carry cholesterol from the liver to the cells of various tissues, where it is used to make cell membranes and certain hormones. For years, medical researchers have known that the cholesterol being deposited in the arteries (atherosclerosis) is the cholesterol attached to LDLs. In contrast, the major function of HDLs is to clear unneeded cholesterol from the tissues and return it to the liver to be excreted. Although their role is not clearly established, HDLs are thought to prevent cholesterol from depositing on the inner walls of the arteries, thus thwarting the process of atherosclerosis. In other words, evidence is accumulating that people who have high levels of HDL cholesterol in their blood tend to be relatively free of heart disease whereas those with high LDL levels are more likely to suffer heart attacks. Many researchers believe that HDL cholesterol is a powerful predictor of coronary artery disease. In addition, research data strongly indicate that middle-aged runners tend to have higher levels of HDL than nonactive people, as well as lower levels of LDL. Such evidence

TABLE 11.1 Cholesterol and the Risk of Heart Disease	
Risk Factor	Risk Level
Total Cholesterol	
<180 mg/dl	Desirable level
180–200 mg/dl	Borderline risk
>200 mg/dl	High risk
High-Density Lipoprotein	
>45 mg/dl	Desirable level
35–45 mg/dl	Borderline risk
<35 mg/dl	High risk
Low-Density Lipoprotein	
<130 mg/dl	Desirable level
130–160 mg/dl	Borderline risk
>160 mg/dl	High risk

makes a strong case for vigorous exercise as a preventive measure in coronary heart disease. Table 11.1 summarizes the relationship between total cholesterol, HDL, and LDL and the risk for heart disease.

Triglycerides are "true" fat particles and represent 95 percent of the total fats stored in the body. In recent years, the triglycerides in the blood have been measured to provide an index of the number of fatty particles floating around in the bloodstream. When excessive amounts of carbohydrates (sugar and starches) are consumed but not used for energy, the excess is turned into fats (triglycerides) and stored. Likewise any saturated fat not readily used is stored. Triglycerides are the main free-floating fat in the bloodstream. Thus, when these fats are not used for immediate energy, the excess is stored within fat cells situated throughout the body—in the abdomen, thighs, arms, chin, and so on. These fats also appear to be associated with atherosclerosis and, like cholesterol, can be lowered by weight loss, diet restrictions, and regular exercise. In fact, research has shown dramatic drops of triglyceride levels with endurance exercise. A diet high in sugar tends to result in high triglyceride levels, and daily consumption of alcohol may lead to elevated triglycerides. The normal range of triglycerides is 10 to 150 mg/dl. Many active people fall well below the 100 mg/dl value.

A 1976 study of the dietary habits, blood lipid levels, and degree of fatness for over 3,000 people in a Michigan community implied that the degree of fatness in an individual was a more obvious determinant of high blood fats than the diet. The authors cautioned that the results of the study do not mean that diet and lipid levels are unrelated. They suggested, rather, that attaining and maintaining a desirable body weight can help prevent and control hyperlipidemia (high blood fats) in the general population. This study and the current research data, which suggest that endurance activities such as walking and running increase HDLs in the blood and reduce LDLs, point to exercise as an important means of preventing heart disease.

Inactivity

Sedentary living is increasingly recognized as a risk factor in heart disease. A recent published review from the Centers for Disease Control in Atlanta supported the contention that regular physical activity appears to serve as a protective mechanism against heart disease. Although inactivity is classified as a lesser influence when compared with the well-known primary risk factors—high levels of blood fat, high blood pressure, and smoking—exercise activity can be the "positive do" that helps control these three major risk factors. People who are active tend to have lower cholesterol and normal blood pressure and most likely don't smoke. In addition, fit people do not have excessive body fat, tend to be able to handle stress more easily, and quite often are more in tune with good eating habits. Thus your approach should be positive—*do exercise*—rather than negative—don't eat this, don't drink that, don't worry, and so on.

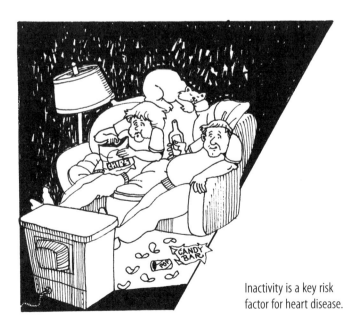

Inactivity is a key risk factor for heart disease.

Active people tend to be able to handle other aspects of their health in a more positive way.

Diabetes

Quite often, diabetes is a hereditary disease, especially when it appears at an early age. **Diabetes** is the inability of the body to break down or properly use sugar in the cells due to a malfunction of the insulin mechanism. **Insulin** is a hormone that controls the rate of entry of glucose (sugar) into the cells. People with diabetes have a high incidence of atherosclerosis. Additionally the severity of coronary heart disease is greater, the death rate is higher, and the incidence of premature heart attack is increased. Women with diabetes have a coronary death rate more than six times that of nondiabetic women. In other words, diabetes negates the protection from coronary heart disease that young women normally enjoy. The actual connection between diabetes and heart disease is not known. One theory suggests that diabetes results in increased fat deposits in the arteries. Again diet management is crucial. If your family has a history of diabetes, you should discuss this with your physician to determine if routine screening for diabetes is necessary.

Research findings continue to suggest that regular vigorous physical activity is beneficial for individuals with diabetes because it helps to clear sugars and fats from the blood. Exercise lowers the blood glucose without the use of insulin. In fact, researchers have found that diabetics who exercise for 30 or more minutes daily have shown as much as 30 to 40 percent reduction in the need for insulin.

Obesity

Obesity, or a condition of excessive fat, is one disease that is clearly evident in our society. The number of overfat persons in the United States has increased 25 percent in the past 20 years. Although estimates vary, children clearly are more overfat today than in past years. National statistics suggest that 35 to 50 percent of all middle-aged Americans are overfat. The high correlation of obesity with high blood pressure and other circulatory diseases underscores the seriousness of being overfat.

Recent research suggests that the way fat is distributed in the body may be an important indicator of heart disease risk. For example, a waist-to-hip ratio greater than 1.0 for men indicates a significantly increased risk; for women, the ratio is 0.8. Thus a man's waist circumference should not exceed his hip measurement. A woman's waist circumference should be 80 percent or less of her hip measurement.

The health problems of an obese person may not be caused by the overweight condition, but rather be linked with a disorder such as heart disease. For example, some individuals with high blood pressure are obese, and a substantial weight loss may lower their blood pressure. Also, due to the consumption of too much food, especially saturated fats, the fat levels in the blood tend to be high. A high concentration of fats in the blood correlates with the presence of atherosclerosis and increases the risk of coronary disease.

During physical work, obesity imposes an increased load on the heart and limits exercise tolerance. Obesity is a health hazard. Although it may not cause heart disease, it does increase the risk for otherwise healthy people. This alone justifies weight reduction. Chapter 10 gives suggestions for combining a nutritious diet with regular vigorous exercise for a lifetime of successful weight management.

Stress

In today's world, it is impossible to live without stress. But excessive amounts of stress over time may create health problems. In the past, researchers typically focused on the possible relationship between one's personal daily stress and coronary heart disease risk. Few researchers bothered to examine the influence of mental and emotional processes on the health of the heart. Two who have are Drs. Meyer Friedman and Ray H. Rosenman. They linked what they term **Type A behavior** with coronary heart disease. They describe this behavior as a complex of emotional reactions to environmental and societal agents that force people to live and work continually faster. They strongly believe that these chronic emotional upsets lead to excessive biochemical changes in the body, such as increased cholesterol levels, that are detrimental to the heart. A sense of "time urgency," a chronic incessant struggle to achieve

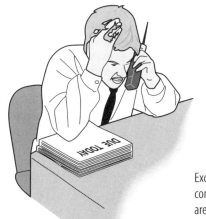

Excessive competitive drive and a compulsion about meeting deadlines are Type A characteristics.

WAY OF LIFE
Psychological Benefits of Exercise

- Enhanced mental energy
- Increased concentration
- Greater self-confidence
- Improved self-esteem

- Enhanced ability to relax
- More positive and enthusiastic outlook on life

more in less time, a demonstration of free-floating hostility, and a tendency to compete aggressively with others are the key Type A characteristics found in many individuals suffering from coronary disease. A research study disclosed that 70 percent of a group of coronary-stricken men exhibited characteristics of "excessive competitive drive and an urgency for meeting deadlines." According to the authors, reducing Type A behavior is a key factor in preventing a heart attack.

Based on our own experiences in conducting exercise programs, we strongly believe that participation in vigorous rhythmical exercise, as recommended throughout this book, has great potential for offsetting some of the tensions and mental stresses characteristic of Type A behavior. Much has been written about the psychological benefits of exercise, specifically running. More and more fitness experts are now addressing the stress reduction benefits of exercise as well. Enhanced mental energy, increased concentration, greater self-confidence, improved self-esteem, and enhanced ability to relax are some of the many benefits attributed to regular fitness exercise. In fact, many psychiatrists now use exercise as a key part of the therapy for their patients.

Increasing numbers of people are discovering a greater sense of mental well-being through regular physical activity. Testimonies of better sleep and improved health are quite common among active people. Although the health benefits of exercise are empirically proven, as you become more active, you may find that the good feeling of being fit is the most important benefit. A positive and enthusiastic outlook on life may go a long way in preventing some stress-related disorders. For more information on managing stress, see Chapter 12.

Cardiac Rehabilitation

In recent years, there have been major medical advances in the management of heart and blood vessel disease. Modern cardiology has expanded to include sophisticated methods for the detection and quantification of cardiovascular diseases. Also, new medical techniques in areas such as heart surgery and new

- Avoid smoking.
- Avoid second-hand smoke.
- Have your blood pressure checked at least once a year.
- Exercise regularly—three to five times per week.
- Reduce your saturated fat intake.
- Reduce your dietary cholesterol.
- Learn to manage stress.

drugs for protecting the diseased heart have produced impressive results. Just as impressive is the more aggressive approach in managing patients after either open-heart surgery or a heart attack. Innovative exercise programs have become an integral part of the rehabilitative process. Broadly defined, **cardiac rehabilitation** encompasses all the measures that serve to restore and maintain a heart patient's optimal physiological, psychological, sociological, educational, and vocational status. The role of exercise has been shown to be a key factor in this multifaceted program. Exercise not only helps restore the physical functions of the body but also enhances psychological, social, and spiritual qualities. Progressively stimulating endurance exercise as a safe means for heart disease therapy is gaining wide acceptance.

Although these rehabilitation efforts are helping patients to achieve a capacity to live a meaningful and active life, the major emphasis in controlling heart disease should be on prevention. *Prevention should begin at birth through the formation of good nutritional and exercise habits.* Per-Olaf Astrand, a famed Swedish medical doctor and physiologist, asserts that because there is so much evidence on the effectiveness of exercise for developing a healthy heart, people should pursue a systematic physical fitness training program. He emphasizes that training the oxygen transport system (the heart, lungs, and circulation) is very important not only as a preventive measure but as a treatment for those afflicted with atherosclerotic diseases.

Physical Activity and Coronary Heart Disease

Several early studies also demonstrated a relationship between levels of physical activity and the incidence of cardiovascular disease. The first study, and one of the largest, was done in London by J. N. Morris and his medical research team over 40 years ago. The team studied 30,000 men employed by the London Transit System, comparing inactive workers (the bus drivers) with active workers (the conductors who walked up and down the double-decker buses). They discovered that the presumably less active bus drivers had many more coronaries than the more active conductors. Morris followed up by studying 10,000 London postal workers. Again the active mail carriers had a lesser incidence of heart attacks than the inactive clerical workers. Although these studies had methodological flaws, they were the first to indicate a relationship between inactivity and a possible risk for heart disease.

The Irish Brothers Study

More than a decade ago, a nine-year study of 575 pairs of brothers born in Ireland was carried out by Harvard's School of Public Health and the School of Medicine at Trinity College, Dublin. One of each pair had remained in Ireland while the other had immigrated to the Boston area. The strictest scientific methods were employed to eliminate extraneous factors.

The researchers had a surprising conclusion: The hearts of the Irishmen, whether rural or urban, were healthier than those of their Boston kinsmen. The Irish brothers had lower blood pressure and lower levels of cholesterol in their bloodstreams. The most astonishing fact was that the Irish brothers ate 400 to 500 more calories each day and had a higher percentage of animal fat in their daily diets than the Americans. Despite their diet, however, they weighed less and had less skinfold fat, as well as lower cholesterol levels. The smoking and drinking habits of both were very similar. Then why were the hearts of the Irish healthier than those of the American brothers? The Irish brothers were generally physically active while their American counterparts were generally sedentary. Physical activity, the researchers concluded, gave the Irish brothers their good health and good hearts.

Other Epidemiological Studies

Dr. Ralph Paffenbarger of the University of California at Berkeley has been researching levels of physical activity and their relationship to reducing heart attack risk. The results of his long-term study of almost 17,000 Harvard alumni suggest that heart attack risk can be significantly reduced by exercising, but only if the exercise is vigorous and burns substantial amounts of calories. Paffenbarger found that those who exercised casually (burning fewer than 2,000 calories a week) had a 64 percent greater heart attack risk than did those who were more active (burning more than 2,000 calories a week). Vigorous activities such as swimming, running, handball, and cycling were cited as the most desirable activities. Paffenbarger is continuing his study, and future data may give us still more insight into the benefits of physical activity as a protector against heart disease.

A study conducted at the Institute for Aerobics Research in Dallas suggests a relationship between physical fitness and longevity. This eight-year study included over 10,000 men and 3,000 women. Physical fitness was quantified using a maximal graded exercise test on a treadmill. Based on the results of the treadmill tests, the subjects were classified into five levels of physical fitness ranging from least fit to most fit. The research team followed these people to determine how their level of physical fitness related to their death rates. After eight years, the inactive individuals in group 1 (least fit) had a death rate more than three times that of individuals in group 5 (most fit). But the most interesting finding was that the death rate for the inactive group was 2.5 times greater than that for those individuals in group 2 (low fitness) who walked 30 minutes per day. The findings of this study suggest that even a low level of fitness can enhance longevity. Steven Blair, the principal researcher, suggests that a brisk walk of 30 minutes or more each day is sufficient to produce a protective level of fitness. Such fitness levels certainly are attainable by most adults.

Summary

Many factors are correlated with coronary heart disease. We are limited in what we can do about some of these factors, such as heredity, sex, race, and age. Nevertheless, we can do something about the other risk factors, such as diet, obesity, smoking, stress, and inactivity. Physical activity can influence each of these risk factors, and exercise aimed at improving cardiorespiratory fitness can be a key to preventing or reducing death from coronary heart disease.

Coronary artery disease isn't like the measles; there is no protective vaccine you can take. It is a disease that develops slowly and subtly and that reflects one of the dangers of living in a highly competitive but sedentary society. The data relating to physical activity and heart disease strongly suggest that an increase in habitual physical activity is beneficial. The most obvious benefits are in the area of improved quality of life, rather than in longevity. Thus physical activity appears to be a prudent means of enhancing health and improving the quality of one's life while also decreasing the risk for cardiovascular disease.

Exercise programs that are "tailored to the capacity and interest of the individual" can enrich the quality of life and, in combination with other measures (such as adopting a low-fat diet or eliminating smoking), can help reduce coronary risk. Fortunately physicians are now more aware of the importance of promoting and maintaining health through regular exercise. The American Medical Association's Committee on Exercise has declared, "Exercise is the most significant factor contributing to the health of the individual." Although this is certainly a bold statement, its truthfulness is backed by the July 1996 surgeon general's report entitled "Physical Activity and Health" (see Chapter 1). The evidence implicating physical inactivity as a cause of death is no longer merely persuasive; it is conclusive.

Key Words

ARTERIOSCLEROSIS: The advanced stage of atherosclerosis when the arteries become hardened.

ATHEROSCLEROSIS: A condition in which the deposits of fatty substances on the inner walls of the arteries build up, narrowing the blood vessels.

CARDIAC REHABILITATION: The management of patients after open-heart surgery or heart attack through a program of exercise and other related interventions to restore their capacity to live meaningful and healthy lives.

CHOLESTEROL: The waxy, fattylike substance that functions as a building block in forming compounds that are vital to body functions. It is produced in the body and is also obtained by eating foods of animal origin. Elevated levels of cholesterol in the blood have been associated with an increased risk of heart and blood vessel disease.

CORONARY HEART DISEASE: The impairment of the coronary arteries to deliver blood due to a buildup of cholesterol and associated fatty substances on the inner portion of the artery walls.

DIABETES: A chronic disorder of glucose (sugar) metabolism due to a disturbance in the normal insulin mechanism.

DIASTOLIC BLOOD PRESSURE: The lowest force exerted by the arterial blood flow against the walls of the vessels.

HIGH-DENSITY LIPOPROTEIN (HDL) CHOLESTEROL: One of the major classes of lipoprotein, often referred to as HDL cholesterol. High levels of HDL cholesterol are associated with increased protection against heart disease.

HYPERTENSION: A higher-than-normal blood pressure, usually defined as any systolic pressure at or above 140 mmHg and/or a diastolic pressure at or above 90 mmHg.

INSULIN: A hormone that controls the rate of glucose entry into cells.

LIPIDS: Fats, or fatlike substances, such as fatty acids, triglycerides, and cholesterol.

LIPOPROTEIN: A type of protein that carries cholesterol and triglycerides in the bloodstream.

LOW-DENSITY LIPOPROTEIN (LDL) CHOLESTEROL: A carrier of large amounts of fat and cholesterol from the liver, where they are made, to the tissues of the body. This is the cholesterol that accumulates in the arteries and leads to clogged arteries.

MYOCARDIAL INFARCTION: Death of part of the heart muscle (myocardium) caused by an interruption of the blood supply to the area; also called a heart attack.

RISK: The possibility or chance that something will happen. In health, it is often expressed in degrees of danger.

SYSTOLIC BLOOD PRESSURE: The greatest force exerted by the arterial blood flow against the walls of the vessels.

TYPE A BEHAVIOR: Behaviors such as an excessive competitive drive and a sense of urgency about time that tend to predispose one to heart disease.

A Way of Life Library

Barry, F., and B. Swinney. *Make the Change for a Healthy Heart.* Colorado Springs, CO: Fall River Press, 1995.

Bouchard, C., R. J. Shephard, and T. Stephens, eds. *Physical Activity, Fitness and Health.* Champaign, IL: Human Kinetics, 1994.

Goor, R., and N. Goor. *Eater's Choice: A Food Lover's Guide to Lower Cholesterol.* New York: Houghton Mifflin, 1995.

Kavanagh, T. *The Healthy Heart Program.* Toronto: Van Nostrand Reinhold, 1980.

CHAPTER 12

Related Health and Fitness Issues

This chapter deals with selected topics associated with being physically active. We discuss stress and the use of exercise in its management. We touch on ways to avoid injuries during a vigorous exercise program and examine the effects of exercise on pregnancy, menstruation, and amenorrhea. We discuss exercising in the heat, in the cold, at altitude, and in polluted air conditions, suggesting precautions for dealing with these conditions. We also examine the dangers of using drugs to enhance physical performance and the effects of using caffeine, alcohol, tobacco, anabolic steroids, and the so-called recreational drugs. Finally, we look at lower-back pain and present methods for reducing your risk of this very common ailment.

As you read this chapter, keep these statements in mind:

- A regular fitness program is an effective tool for coping with stress.
- Common sense can help you avoid exercise-induced injuries.
- Mild to moderate exercise during pregnancy is safe for most women and can benefit them both physiologically and psychologically.
- Exercising in high heat and humidity can cause serious problems and requires precautions.
- Frostbite and loss of body temperature are two dangers associated with below-freezing workouts. Nevertheless, exercising in cold weather can be safe and very invigorating.
- Exercise presents a viable alternative to "recreational" drug use.

Managing Stress

Stress is a normal part of everyone's day. It is common to hear people complain about the stress they are under. **Stress** is defined as a mental, emotional, and physical response resulting from an event or some real or imagined factor in your life. Such stressors force your body into a physiological or psychological state of imbalance. Whether the stress is related to your job, your studies, or your social life, too much stress over time can affect your health. Helping people learn to cope effectively with these daily stresses has been a concern of health and medical professionals in recent years. Regular exercise, when practiced in a reasonable manner, has been an effective tool for many people to relieve stress.

Dr. Hans Selye, a world-famous Canadian scientist, described stress as the nonspecific response of the body to any demand placed on it. The term *nonspecific* refers to the body reacting in a similar manner regardless of the type of event that led to the stress. Selye identified two types of stress. **Eustress** is stress that can enhance performance and healthy living; **distress** is stress that can be harmful and unpleasant. If distress goes unchecked or gets out of control, the long-term consequences can include serious health problems such as hypertension, heart disease, depression, headaches, insomnia, and even menstrual irregularities. Also, dependency behaviors such as overeating and smoking tend to relate to unresolved stress. In short, continued distress or unresolved stress can diminish your quality of life.

Your personal expectations and those of your family often elicit some unpleasant pressures. No one is immune to failure. Learning how to manage your everyday life is important for you to succeed. So how do you cope? Being able to recognize stressors is the key to maintaining emotional and physiological

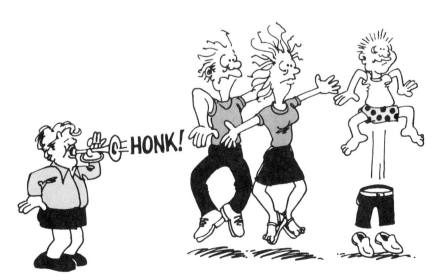

Everyday stresses may be harmful to one's health.

TABLE 12.1 Symptoms of Distress	
Anger, hostility	Loss of appetite
Depression	Muscular aches (neck, shoulders, back)
Frustration	Poor concentration
Headaches	Restlessness, pacing
High blood pressure	Stomach pains (possible ulcers, digestive disorders)
Increase in appetite	
Insomnia (inability to sleep)	Unusual fatigue

stability. You can learn to identify the symptoms associated with stress and implement strategies of stress management.

Symptoms of Stress

A moderate degree of stress is normal. However, when stressful events increase, tension and anxiety begin to surface. Unfortunately many sources of stress are beyond your control. Sitting in congested traffic, waiting in line at the store, and trying to meet work or school deadlines are just a few examples of unavoidable stresses. Stress can be cumulative, and if you ignore it, over time it can take its toll on your body. For example, prolonged tension can lead to headaches, backaches, and digestive disorders, to name a few. Uncontrolled stress can elevate blood pressure, eventually leading to a heart attack. Even your eating and sleeping habits can be negatively affected by stress. Table 12.1 lists some common symptoms of distress. Although the list is not all-inclusive, the key is to recognize these symptoms and take steps to alleviate the stressful events. Finding time to exercise or to relax are ways to manage your stress.

The Role of Exercise in Stress Management

Regular exercise is one of the best ways to cope with the tensions and frustrations of daily living. Exercise reduces stress by decreasing muscular tension and serving as a diversion from the day's events. Many exercisers report how invigorating a workout makes them feel—their muscles are relaxed and they feel calm after a workout. In fact, many people use midday exercise as a welcome break from daily stress. Exercising late in the afternoon or early evening also can help dissipate the built-up stresses of the day. Most health, fitness, and medical professionals agree that exercise is an excellent way to reduce feelings of anger, anxiety, frustration and aggression.

TABLE 12.2
Progressive Muscle Relaxation

1. Wrinkle your forehead and make a face. Feel the tension. Hold, then relax. Repeat.
2. Close your eyes tightly. Feel the tension. Hold, then relax, leaving your eyes closed. Repeat.
3. Press your teeth together. Feel the tension. Hold, then relax. Repeat.
4. Slowly bring your head to your chest, pushing your chin into your chest. Feel the tension in your neck. Hold, then relax. Repeat.
5. Slowly push your head backwards. Feel the tension in the back of your neck. Hold, then relax. Repeat.
6. Raise your shoulders toward your ears as far as possible. Feel the tension. Hold, then relax. Repeat.
7. Place your arms flat on the floor, palms up. Push hard with your forearms against the floor. Feel the tension on your arms. Hold, then relax. Repeat.
8. Bend your elbows, bringing both hands to your shoulders. Tighten your forearms hard against your biceps. Feel the tension in your biceps. Hold, then relax. Repeat.
9. With your arms at the side of your body, clench both fists. Feel the tension. Hold, then relax. Repeat.
10. Suck in your stomach by contracting your abdominals. Flatten your lower back to the floor. Feel the tension in your abdominal muscles. Hold, then relax. Repeat.
11. Tighten your buttocks. Feel the tension. Hold, then relax. Repeat.
12. Contract one thigh by straightening your leg and slowly raising it off the floor a couple of inches. Hold it and feel the tension. Then return your leg to the floor. Relax. Repeat with the other leg. Contract and relax each leg again.
13. Push or force your heels down against the floor. Feel the tension on the back of your thighs and calves. Hold, then relax. Repeat.
14. Bend your feet toward your upper body. Feel the tension in your feet and lower front leg muscles. Hold, then relax. Repeat.
15. Point your feet and toes downward and away from your upper body. Feel the tension in the arches, calves, and Achilles tendons. Hold, then relax. Repeat.

Source: Adapted from Edmund Jacobson, *Anxiety and Tension Control* (Philadelphia: Lippincott, 1964).

Relaxation Techniques

Relaxation techniques have long been used to help people cope with stress. One technique, **progressive muscle relaxation,** has been effectively used to reduce muscular tension; Table 12.2 outlines the specific techniques involved. These relaxation exercises should be conducted in a quiet and comfortable room. Stretch out on the floor, face up, with a pillow under your knees. Contract and relax the various muscle groups in a sequential manner, tightening a muscle group for 5 to 7 seconds and then allowing your muscles to relax or go totally limp. Allow 20 minutes to perform the complete sequence listed in Table 12.2.

Avoiding Injuries

Exercise obviously has many benefits, but it can also lead to injuries. Fortunately common sense can help you avoid injuries. For instance, many injuries are simply the result of overuse—doing too much too soon. This is why we urge you to follow the recommendations described for each specific exercise mode. Your body needs time to adjust gradually to the suggested exercise work loads. The best plan is to progressively increase work loads in small increments. Some enthusiastic beginners, however, may be tempted to ignore our suggestions and increase the duration or intensity of their workouts on their own. At a beginner's level, doing too much too soon can lead to injury. Following the "10-percent rule" (see Chapter 5) will lessen your chances of injury.

Expect some muscle and joint soreness during the first few weeks of a new activity or if you speed up your program. These discomforts are the result of new demands on your muscles, and may occur even though you have been active in another fitness activity or a sport. This initial discomfort should not hinder your daily progress. In fact, an "active recovery" in which you keep moving steadily is important in overcoming muscle soreness.

Even though studies have failed to conclusively show a relationship between warming up and injury prevention, it is a good idea to include a warm-up period in your program. Prevention beats injury every time! We do know that stretching, especially following your cool-down, improves flexibility. This is particularly helpful as your workouts get progressively more vigorous.

Instructors who lead group exercise sessions, such as dance aerobics or step aerobics, should offer some guidance on injury avoidance. However, many instructors are not fully qualified to give you this information. Part of your responsibility as a fitness consumer is to participate only in exercise classes led by educated and certified instructors. A degree in physical education or exercise science is highly desirable. The most recognized and recommended certifications are those provided by the American College of Sports Medicine, the American Council on Exercise (ACE), or the Aerobics and Fitness Association of America (AFAA). To locate a certified instructor near you, contact any of these organizations.

Women and Exercise

Millions of women have been caught up in the health and physical fitness boom. This interest has led to more research on the relationship between exercise and such women's health issues as menstruation, pregnancy, and amenorrhea. Because men and women clearly are more similar than different in their responses to exercise, all of the information provided earlier in this book applies to both sexes. However, this section highlights areas in which there truly are gender differences and in which modifications in a woman's training program might be warranted.

Menstruation

The effects of exercise on **menstruation,** and vice versa, have been misunderstood for years. Not long ago, girls commonly were excused from physical education class during their menstrual periods. Coaches, physical educators, and physicians felt that this was the proper thing to do. In some schools, this practice still occurs.

Today females are much more likely to continue exercising during their menstrual periods. In fact, females have won Olympic medals during every phase of the menstrual cycle. Scientific evidence supports the view that the normal routine of life should not be interrupted during menstruation. Also, there is no evidence that vigorous fitness activity causes the menstrual disorder **dysmenorrhea,** which is painful or difficult menstruation. In fact, although we are not quite sure why, many women find that physical activity actually helps ease cramping and premenstrual tension. Thus many females have come to rely on their workouts for some measure of relief.

Amenorrhea

Because the menstrual period is a normal physiological function, most females can continue regular vigorous exercise regardless of where they are in their cycles. However, some extremely active female athletes have reported cessation of their menstrual periods, or **secondary amenorrhea.** The causes of amenorrhea and its long-term consequences are not fully understood. Current research suggests that amenorrhea may be related to acute effects of stress (both physiological and psychological), to low levels of body fat, or to the levels of the circulating hormones. The incidence of amenorrhea tends to be greater among females who train daily for many hours and less among those who work at higher intensities for shorter periods. Amenorrhea is common in females involved with gymnastics, long-distance running, and ballet. Nevertheless many lean athletes who train intensely for competition menstruate regularly.

In the past, many amenorrheic athletes did not mind the absence of their periods and simply decreased workout frequency, duration, and/or intensity to become regular again. Medical doctors generally believed that this phenomenon was no cause for alarm and that amenorrhea was possibly an appropriate response of the body to heavy exercise training. However, more recent research on amenorrheic athletes has discovered significantly lower-than-normal bone densities, possibly due to lower levels of circulating estrogen. The bone densities of amenorrheic athletes may fall to such low levels that they resemble the bones of postmenopausal women. Low bone density leads to a condition known as osteoporosis, which results in brittle bones that are prone to fracture. Once fractures have occurred, a full recovery is unlikely. But new drugs that might reverse the effects of osteoporosis once the damage has been done hold great promise. Still, the best treatment for osteoporosis is actually prevention. Therefore coaches and their amenorrheic athletes need to take the condition seriously and consider all lifestyle and training changes necessary to prevent or reverse amenorrhea, rather than simply ignore it.

Pregnancy and Childbirth

Women today are more likely than ever to continue to exercise throughout pregnancy. They feel better physiologically and psychologically, recognizing that pregnancy is a state of being, not a disability. Because of the interest in exercise and pregnancy, much new information has been uncovered on maternal and fetal responses to exercise. Reviews of the literature reveal that even though a pregnant mother's heart rate increases during exercise, there are no adverse effects on either the mother or the fetus. Additionally recent research has found no evidence of fetal distress or abnormalities due to a mother's increased core temperature during exercise. Previous guidelines for exercise and pregnancy were updated at a 1994 conference of the American College of Obstetricians and Gynecologists. These guidelines differentiate between women who exercise regularly and become pregnant and women who begin exercising after they become pregnant. In general, already-exercising women should continue their training while women just starting to exercise should consult with their physician first. Also, these newly exercising women should begin with low-intensity, nonimpact activities like cycling and swimming. Any woman considering becoming pregnant would be wise to *develop optimal physical fitness prior to conception and maintain that level throughout pregnancy.*

At rest, a pregnant woman's heart rate tends to be 15 to 20 beats higher than normal. Therefore standard formulas for target heart-rate ranges are inaccurate. In the past, pregnant women were advised to keep their exercise heart rates at 140 beats per minute or less. This recommendation was conservative and did not take into account age, previous fitness levels, or previous target heart-rate ranges. The updated guidelines now encourage pregnant women to exercise at mild to moderate intensities at least three times per week. A pregnant woman should listen to her body's response and modify exercise intensity according to any symptoms experienced. She should stop exercising when fatigue sets in, not at the point of exhaustion. Many physically fit women can continue weight-bearing exercise like walking, running, and aerobics at their prepregnancy intensities. However, non-weight-bearing activities like rowing and swimming may reduce the risk of injury while increasing exercise adherence throughout the pregnancy.

Although the restrictions on exercise during pregnancy are relatively few, some modifications may be warranted. For instance, a pregnant woman's center of gravity shifts as her body changes shape and size. Physical activities that require a lot of balance (like skiing) may not be appropriate, particularly in the third trimester. Obviously any exercise that has even the slightest potential for abdominal trauma should be avoided. Also pregnant women should not exercise in the supine position after the first trimester. This position is accompanied by a decrease in cardiac output, which is the amount of blood pumped per minute. The decreased cardiac output is a direct result of the weight of the fetus pressing down on the main veins returning blood from the lower extremities. This frequently leads to light-headedness or fainting and decreased blood flow to the fetus. Furthermore pregnant women should avoid standing motionless for prolonged periods of time (such as waiting in line for the stair climbing machine at the fitness center). Finally pregnant women should take every precaution not to become overheated, which means staying well hydrated and choosing clothing and an environment that allows for dissipation of heat.

It's still unclear whether exercising during pregnancy makes labor and delivery easier. Regular exercise during pregnancy does help control excess weight gain and reduces the time that it takes a woman to return to her prepregnancy body composition. Possessing a high level of cardiorespiratory endurance helps a pregnant woman sustain the effort of delivery. A high level of muscular strength and endurance, particularly in the abdominal muscles, better enables a woman to bear down and push during delivery. Following childbirth, overall muscular strength and endurance allows a woman to pick up and carry her baby without fatiguing. In summary, maintaining an optimal fitness level during pregnancy remains as important as during any other stage in life.

The new mother's body normally take four to six weeks following childbirth to return to prepregnancy conditions. A physically fit woman may recover more quickly. Regardless, the prepregnancy routines should be resumed gradually. It is important for a woman to listen to her body and to train based on her capabilities, not on the calendar.

Amidst all this good news regarding pregnancy and exercise, there certainly are situations in which exercise is contraindicated or the standard guidelines need modifying. These include the following:

- Pregnancy-induced hypertension
- Preterm rupture of the membrane
- Preterm labor during the prior or current pregnancy
- Incompetent cervix
- Persistent second- to third-trimester bleeding
- Intrauterine growth retardation

A pregnant woman's close communication with her obstetrician is highly recommended and especially important if she is physically active and/or prone to any of these conditions.

Environmental Conditions

You need to be aware of environmental factors that can affect your workouts. This section will briefly highlight how to deal with air pollution, heat, cold, and high altitude during your training sessions.

Exercising in Polluted Air

Exercising outdoors can be a refreshing and invigorating aspect of your training program, especially after spending hours indoors. Unfortunately air pollution is the one environmental factor that cannot always be surmounted. The pollutants most often identified as having possible detrimental effects on the body are carbon monoxide, ozone, and sulfur dioxide. Carbon monoxide comes primarily from automobile exhaust and cigarettes. Large amounts of carbon monoxide in the air reduce the oxygen-carrying capacity of the blood. Ozone and sulfur dioxide are known to cause constriction of the airway tubes in your lungs, making it difficult to breathe. Wheezing, coughing, and other lung-related problems can occur. Not only will exercising in polluted air hurt your performance, but over time it may have detrimental effects on your health.

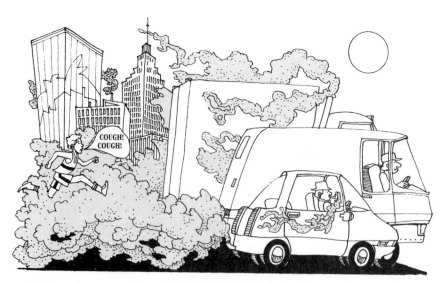

Inhaling carbon monoxide hurts performance and may have detrimental effects on your health.

If you live in an area that frequently experiences a high air pollution index or has air safety alerts, check before exercising outdoors. On a poor air quality day, exercisers are at a higher health risk than the general population because of having to breathe in larger amounts of air continuously for 30 to 45 minutes. Either have an indoor alternative or wait until a safer time of day when alerts are withdrawn. Exercising in the early morning when pollution is the lowest is a good idea.

Exercising in the Cold

An obvious danger associated with cold-weather workouts is rapid loss of body heat. A rapid drop in body temperature leads to violent shivering and impairment in coodination and the ability to think clearly. This loss of body temperature, called **hypothermia,** is potentially fatal. The risk of hypothermia is greatest when you are out in the cold for many hours and when winds are high or the weather is damp. If you get wet or injured and can't move well enough to stay warm, hypothermia can become a reality. This is why it is good practice to work out with a friend.

Another danger of exercising in cold environments is frostbite, which is freezing of the skin. Symptoms of frostbite include numbness and white discoloration of the skin. Your hands, ears, toes, and face are particularly vulnerable at temperatures below 20°F. Due to its cooling effect on exposed skin, the wind can drastically increase your risk for frostbite. Today most weather updates give you the **windchill factor,** which is based on the wind speed and temperature. Before exercising in the cold, pay attention to the windchill rather than the actual temperature. Whenever the windchill index is minus 20°F or below, you probably should not put yourself at risk by exercising outdoors.

When exercising in a cold environment, expect to spend a bit more time warming up. Your body temperature may take slightly longer to elevate, so be patient. Contrary to what some people think, your lungs will not freeze when you are exercising in the cold. However, your throat may stay more comfortable during cold-weather workouts if you wear a face mask or a bandana around your mouth and nose.

Exercising in the cold requires dressing properly. Most people, believe it or not, overdress. Even in cold weather, exercise raises the body temperature significantly. As a rule of thumb, you know you are not overdressed if you feel slightly chilled when you step outside. If you are comfortable even before you begin to exercise, you are probably overdressed.

In cold weather, you want to wear several layers of loose-fitting, thin clothing. This allows you to trap the body heat you generate but also to remove one or more layers if you begin to get too warm. Generally your first layer should be made of material that wicks moisture away from your skin, such as polypropylene. Succeeding layers can be a T-shirt, a turtleneck, a wool sweater, and,

---

WAY OF LIFE
Working Out Safely in the Cold

- Know the windchill factor before you go outside to work out.
- In severe cold weather with a windchill below minus 20° F, exercise indoors or skip it for a day.

- Dress in layers, and be sure to cover your ears and head.
- Avoid slippery roads and heavy traffic areas.
- Work out with a friend in case of a problem.

---

if necessary, a windbreaker jacket as the outer layer. As you get warm, you might remove one or more layers and tie the arms around your waist. At the risk of sounding like your mother, don't forget a hat, at least at the start of your workout, because a lot of body heat is lost through the head. Also, because your hands and fingers are "second-rate citizens" during exercise and don't always receive enough blood in the cold, you should wear light gloves or even socks over your hands. They can easily be stuffed up your sleeves if they are no longer needed.

Perhaps the greatest obstacle to outdoor exercise in the cold is ice. Shoe, tire, and even ski undersurfaces are not usually designed for traction on such a slippery surface, so trying to negotiate a workout on a sheet of ice can be frustrating and dangerous. Ask most fitness enthusiasts about their experiences with ice, and you likely will hear painful accounts of normally upright exercise postures suddenly becoming horizontal. You can take all the precautions to prevent frostbite and hypothermia only to fall on an icy road. Also avoid heavy traffic areas. The automobiles with which you are sharing the road also have limited traction. Use good sense and consider an indoor alternative on extremely icy days.

Exercising in the Heat

As dangerous as cold-weather exercising can be, heat and humidity must be respected to an even greater extent. When the air temperature gets above your skin temperature (generally greater than 90°F), your body gains heat from the environment rather than loses it. Thus the primary mechanism for cooling becomes the evaporation of sweat. If both the temperature and relative humidity are high, your body's ability to cool itself is severely compromised because the sweat will not readily evaporate. These conditions can cause your internal

WAY OF LIFE
Working Out Safely in Heat and Humidity

- Know the temperature and relative humidity before you go outside to work out.
- Drink water prior to, during, and after exercise.
- Monitor your exercise heart rate carefully.
- Wear appropriate clothing that allows heat to escape from your body.

- Consider exercising during a cooler part of the day.
- Exercise indoors in air-conditioned facilities on extreme days.
- Know the signs of heat illness and ways to deal with it.

body temperature to rise, possibly leading to heat illness, heat exhaustion, or even heat stroke.

The hot-weather equivalent of the windchill factor is the heat index, which is based on temperature and relative humidity. The relative humidity gives an indication of how readily the air absorbs moisture. High relative humidity indicates that the air is already saturated with water, so evaporation of sweat is hindered. Before exercising in the heat, pay attention to the heat index rather than the actual temperature. Even at relatively cool temperatures, if the humidity is high, our bodies can overheat. On days with a high heat index, train indoors or during the cooler part of the day.

If you are not accustomed to exercising in a warm climate, you need to give yourself time to acclimate. Take at least 10 days, decreasing speed (work load) and possibly duration of your training until your body's thermostat resets. Follow your heart rate closely, and expect to slow down on hotter days to stay within your target heart-rate range. Most fitness exercisers have two exercise paces, one for temperate weather and a slightly slower one for hot, humid days. If you exercise on a regular basis, the transition from one season to another should not present a problem.

Dehydration is your worst enemy. It affects your physical performance more than any other factor and can be life-threatening. Drink plenty of water (preferably cool water) before, during, and after exercise in the heat. You cannot rely on your thirst level to indicate whether you need water. Drink about one cup every 15 minutes whether you are thirsty or not. Runners going long distances on a hot, humid day have been known to drive their route beforehand and plant water bottles at regular intervals to remain hydrated. Some people even weigh themselves on a scale prior to exercising in the heat and humidity. After completing their workout, they stand on the scale and drink whatever amount is needed to return themselves to preexercise weight.

Clothing must allow for air circulation and sweat evaporation. Wear clothing that is loose-fitting and light in both color and weight. Cotton or mesh materials are best. Finally don't forget your sun block with an SPF of 15 or greater.

Exercising at Higher Altitudes

For the majority of Americans living near sea level, exercising at high altitudes brings about instant humility. Your cardiorespiratory system has a more difficult time delivering enough oxygen for vigorous activity, and what may have been aerobic exercise at home quickly becomes anaerobic in the mountains. Give yourself five to seven days or longer to become acclimated. In the meantime, use your target heart-rate range and perceived exertion as your guides for exercise intensity. As in hot, humid conditions, expect to perform your workout at a slower pace if you want to stay in your target heart-rate range. Once all your systems have adapted, you should be able to handle your previous work loads. When you are planning to travel to the mountains, arrive in good physical condition. The greater your fitness level, the better you will adjust to high altitude and the more you will enjoy your activities.

Being able to hike or run through the woods during the summer heat, cruise down the ski slopes at high altitude, or cross-country ski on a cold, wintery day are some of the benefits of being in good shape. Although there are potential dangers associated with hot, cold, and high-altitude conditions, you can fully enjoy your workouts by using good judgment and adhering to the guidelines presented in this section. Remember, you can't beat Mother Nature, so be patient and enjoy the variety that different environmental conditions add to your workout.

Lower-Back Pain

Nearly 80 percent of American adults suffer from back pain at some point in their lives. Among common ailments, lower-back pain is second only to headaches. In general, the causes of backaches include poor posture, improper body mechanics, inactivity, and excess body fatness. Excess body fat, particularly concentrated around the abdomen, adds to the postural muscles' work load. In other words, the structures in the spinal region (bone, ligaments, and muscle) may not have enough strength to support the weight of the body.

Common remedies for back pain include heat applications and medications. But such treatments are not directed at the primary cause, which frequently is poor physical fitness. Although serious structural abnormalities such as ruptured vertebral disks cause lower-back pain, they are estimated to account for less than 5 percent of all cases. According to statistics, about 80 percent of back pain cases arise from muscular weakness or inelasticity.

Prevention

The lower portion of the spine is a complicated system of bones (vertebrae), muscles, ligaments, and nerves. The primary function of the bones of the spinal column is to house and protect the spinal cord. Not only does the spine have to support the weight of the upper body, but it must be able to bend, stretch, and twist in any direction. Thus it is more vulnerable to strain and fatigue than other areas of the body.

When you look at your body from the side, the lower back is normally curved inward; it is not straight. Back trouble can occur when the curve becomes accentuated in either direction. Even though millions of people suffer from lower-back pain, it generally can be prevented with proper posture and sensible exercise. Alignment of the spine and pelvis must allow for a natural, mild lower-back curve, with the top of the pelvis not tilted too far forward or backward.

When specific muscle groups are weak and/or inflexible, it is difficult to maintain this correct posture. Abdominals, hip flexors and extensors, and lower-back muscles should be specifically targeted for improvement. For example, weak abdominals are unable to hold the pelvis in neutral alignment with the spine, thus allowing the top of the pelvis to tilt too far forward. This shortens the lower-back and hip flexor muscles and accentuates lower-back curvature. At the other extreme, overcorrecting for an exaggerated lower-back curve or inflexible hip extensors may cause the top of the pelvis to tilt too far backward, leading to a flattened lower back. Prolonged periods of time in either of these unnatural postures leads to pain. The strengthening (see Chapter 7) and flexibility (see Chapter 8) exercises for the abdominal, lower back, and hip flexor and extensor muscles will reduce your risk for back pain by allowing your spine and pelvis to maintain a natural position.

Posture

Chronic fatigue and lower-back muscle strain often result from poor posture. The following simple rules for sleeping, sitting, and standing will help you improve your posture and decrease your risk for lower-back pain.

Sleeping

Incorrect sleeping positions can place a great deal of strain on the back. Sleeping facedown causes your back to arch, especially if you rest your head on a pillow. Sleeping on your back with your legs straight also causes arching. The correct posture for sleeping is on your side, with your hips and knees bent and your head supported by a pillow. Another possibility, although not as practical, is to lie on your back with your knees flexed. Using a pillow under your knees as a support helps.

Sitting

A good basic rule for sitting is to have your knees level with or slightly higher than your hips. When your knees are lower than your hips, your back tends to overarch. Following this rule when driving will also spare your back. In addition, avoid sitting in any one position for long periods of time. Believe it or not, sitting places more strain on the lower back than either the standing or walking positions. Taking frequent breaks and stretching can go a long way to preventing lower-back discomfort.

Standing

Standing is very tiring for your back. As fatigue sets in, your hips begin to sag forward. If you are overfat in your abdominal region, you will suffer further arching due to the additional weight in the front of your body. This postural problem can be solved by elevating either foot. Such measure takes the arch out of the back. The basic rule is that when you stand in one position for a long time, you should flex one of your hips by supporting one foot higher than the other. As long as one hip is flexed, your lower back will tend not to strain forward. (No wonder the old stand-up bars in western saloons always had a footrest running the length of the bar!)

High-heeled shoes also contribute to overarching of the lower back. If you must wear them, you might consider also carrying along a comfortable pair of flat shoes. Wear them whenever walking to and from your car or at lunch time. Minimizing the time you spend in heels will spare your lower back.

Lifting

Improper lifting habits can also lead to serious back problems. There are two key rules for lifting. First, never bend forward without bending your knees. Reaching down to pick up a load with your knees straight places tremendous pressure on the muscles and vertebral disks. When lifting, get as close to the object as possible and squat down, bending at the hips and knees. Looking forward (rather than down), with your lower back as upright as possible, use the large muscles of the legs and hips to help you lift.

Second, be extra careful when lifting or carrying heavy objects. When you lift an object higher than your waist, your hips rotate forward and your back arches to help maintain balance. This places excessive strain on the lower back. Try to store heavy objects on shelves lower than waist height, and ask for help when lifting heavy objects overhead. When carrying heavy objects, hold them against your body at waist level. Doing so minimizes the chances for muscle strain.

Drugs

Drug abuse is a major crisis in America today. National surveys indicate that persons ages 18 to 25 are most likely to use illegal drugs. When a person uses drugs for reasons other than medical treatment, prevention, or pain relief, it is called recreational drug use. The various reasons for recreational drug use include trying to lessen social tensions, creating pleasurable sensations, enhancing physical performance, rebelling against the pressures of society, and/or improving chances of peer acceptance. However, when a drug user's life becomes disrupted by any number of physiological and psychological problems, drug use frequently becomes drug abuse. Drug abuse can interfere with school performance and personal relationships; it can lead to job loss, cut short promising careers, and seriously affect one's physical fitness. In other words, it can ruin lives.

Many drug abusers are not aware they have a problem. They rationalize that they can stop anytime they want. Unfortunately the research shows this is not true in many cases. To determine if you have a potential drug abuse problem, answer the questions in the accompanying Way of Life box. If you answer yes to two or more questions, we urge you to talk to a substance abuse counselor at your nearest medical/health center.

Drug Categories

Drugs are classified according to the physiological effect they have on your body. Here are some of the more common classifications:

- *Stimulants:* These speed up your nervous system and increase alertness and excitability.
- *Depressants:* Also known as tranquilizers or sedatives, these slow down your nervous system and help you to relax.
- *Psychoactives:* These substances alter moods, feelings, and perceptions.

WAY OF LIFE
When to Get Help for a Drug or Alcohol Problem

- Do you take drugs or drink to get ready for social situations?
- Do you take drugs or drink to avoid facing personal problems?
- Do you hide your drinking or drug use from others?
- Do you take drugs and drink when you're alone?
- Do you get annoyed when someone suggests that you drink or take drugs too much?

- *Narcotics:* These powerful painkillers can also cause pleasurable feelings.
- *Inhalants:* These volatile nondrugs produce druglike effects when inhaled; glue and gasoline fall in this category.
- *Designer drugs:* These illegally manufactured drugs tend to mimic controlled substances; generally they are more powerful and dangerous than the drugs they mimic.

Commonly Abused Drugs

In this section, we review the most commonly abused drugs. Caffeine, alcohol, and nicotine are classified as drugs. All are legal and commonly used today in our society. However, all have the potential to be harmful if abused. Anabolic steroids and growth hormones, most often used by strength athletes and bodybuilders, are also a major health concern, as are the recreational drugs, such as cocaine and marijuana.

Caffeine

Caffeine is a stimulant. Millions of people drink or ingest caffeine daily, from cola drinks, chocolate, and, of course, coffee. High doses of caffeine can cause headaches, gastric irritability, insomnia, jitteriness, and irregular heartbeat. The physiological effects of caffeine on exercise and sports performance, particularly those of long duration, are unclear. We do know that caffeine is a

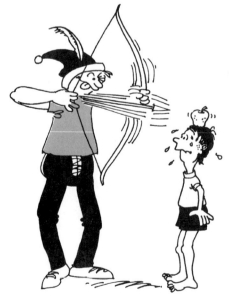

High doses of caffeine can cause jitteriness and irregular heartbeats.

diuretic. Diuretics increase water loss via frequent urination, which can lead to dehydration. Because caffeinated drinks stimulate water loss, they cannot be considered as our daily requirement for water. This is of particular importance for individuals involved in vigorous exercise, because they lose additional water as sweat. Thus paying extra attention to water consumption should be a priority for these people. In fact, for every caffeinated drink they consume, they should drink a comparable amount of water to cancel out the caffeine's effects. Also, anyone consuming large amounts of caffeine prior to outdoor exercise had better plan bathroom locations on their routes! Overall, restricting daily consumption to a couple of cups of coffee or cola drinks allows you to enjoy caffeine without harming your health.

Alcohol

Although socially acceptable, alcohol has probably caused more social, emotional, and physical damage to users and their families than any other drug. People drink to celebrate, to relax, to ease social situations, to feel good, and for a multitude of other reasons. Because alcohol is accepted in society as legal and appropriate, it is important to use it responsibly. This means drinking slowly (not more than one drink per hour), eating when drinking, and, most important, not mixing drinking and driving. Likewise exercise and alchohol are not compatible. Because alchohol acts as a diuretic, like caffeine, consuming it can lead to dehydration. There is no evidence to suggest that alcohol improves exercise or sports performance. In fact, because alcohol impairs balance and coordination, it actually hinders it.

Tobacco

Tobacco products all contain **nicotine,** an addictive substance and a poison. There is nicotine in cigarettes, cigars, pipe tobacco, and the various forms of smokeless tobacco (snuff and chewing tobacco). The use of tobacco is directly or indirectly responsible for a number of health problems and diseases. Cancer of the lungs and the mouth are common diseases resulting from tobacco use. Heart disease and diseases of the peripheral arteries in the body also are attributed to cigarette smoking. Smoking mothers do a disservice to their children. Not only are the chances for complications during pregnancy increased, but rates for pneumonia and bronchitis are significantly higher in children of smoking mothers. Although teenage smoking is on the rise, many adults—especially those who are better educated—are kicking the smoking habit. Those who quit this deadly habit eventually decrease their risk for cancer and early heart disease to the level of a nonsmoker. A bonus is that their clothes and breath no longer smell of tobacco, and food begins to taste better.

Because nicotine is a stimulant, smokers' resting heart rates will be elevated, and depending on when they smoked their last cigarette, so will their exercise heart rates. Smoking also increases airway tube resistance, thus making breathing more difficult. Obviously this has detrimental effects on exercise and sports performance. Isn't it ironic that so many sporting events are sponsored by tobacco companies?

Steroids

Anabolic steroids are powerful drugs that can increase body weight, muscle size, and strength. They are synthetically produced compounds similar in chemical structure to the male hormone testosterone. Anabolic steroids are used medically to treat individuals with certain cancers or with deficient hormone levels. Dosages for these legitimate medical treatments tend to be low, and patients are closely monitored by their doctors. Conversely, for anabolic steroids to be effective in normal individuals, dosages need to be 10 or more times higher than normally prescribed. These high dosages are often associated with side effects ranging from acne to cancer. In fact, over 70 harmful side effects have been identified.

The most pervasive, yet most ignored, side effect is early onset of cardiovascular disease. In addition, anabolic steroids can stop bone growth, resulting in short stature if taken by youngsters or teenagers. In males, the testicles shrink, and impotence and sterility can result. Female users tend to suffer from masculinizing effects such as deepening of the voice and increased facial and body hair. Steroids also can cause depression and violent behavior. And steroid injections have led to infections such as hepatitis (a liver disease) and AIDS. Because of the associated health risks, as well as ethical issues, the use of anabolic steroids is banned in sports by almost every national and international governing body. Furthermore, the sale and/or possession of anabolic steroids is now illegal due to their recent classification as a Category III controlled substance.

"Recreational" Drugs

The most widely used recreational drugs are cocaine and marijuana. Use of these drugs produces feelings of exhilaration, euphoria, and well-being. The effect is rapid, and the high lasts from 5 to 20 minutes for cocaine to 2 to 4 hours for marijuana. After the euphoric feeling subsides, depression often follows. Both drugs have associated complications, with those from cocaine being the most severe. Besides being addictive, cocaine has dramatic and occasionally fatal effects on the nervous system and heart. Neither drug is beneficial with regard to exercise or sports performance, nor do they have a place in healthy lives.

Your quality of life is enhanced when you take control of those factors that either allow you to reach or prohibit you from attaining your potential. Not surprisingly, the quality of life experienced by a drug abuser is at the opposite end of the spectrum from that experienced by a fit and energetic individual. When you choose to eat right and exercise regularly, you also adopt behaviors that build you up, not tear you down. As many fitness "junkies" will tell you, exercise becomes a "positive addiction" that they crave both physiologically and psychologically. Not only does the actual physical movement feel good, but they get hooked on its many benefits as well. Having said that, it is also important to avoid a "negative addiction" to exercise such that you forgo all other life obligations in order to get your workout in. A fitness lifestyle should improve your life, not complicate or destroy it.

Summary

As mentioned previously, we live in a stressful society. A lot of things make us feel good, but many of these things may not be good for us. Unfortunately many people turn to alcohol, tranquilizers, cigarettes, and illegal drugs to offset their daily stresses. Throughout this book, the main theme has been to help you develop a lifestyle that is more consistent with good health. Regular exercise, good nutrition, and relaxation techniques are essential ingredients to health and wellness.

Healthier people tend to handle stressful situations without suffering the harmful and sometimes destructive effects. Physically fit people tend to be more in control of their lives. They live life more fully.

The fitness boom's staying power over the years means it is no longer a fad, but rather a way of life for millions of people. Throughout this period of growth, fitness professionals have developed guidelines for a variety of health- and fitness-related issues. Exercise guidelines have been created in part to help prevent exercise-induced injuries. We have also improved our knowledge of how to exercise under extreme climatic conditions. Likewise, with more women than ever engaging in vigorous exercise, research on issues relating to the female body has expanded tremendously. And we know that there is no place for drug dependence in a healthy lifestyle. The best alternative to the instant gratification that recreational drugs offer is to adopt and maintain an active way of life. Being physically fit means having a body that can function at its optimal efficiency. This translates into the robust health and the availability of excess energy needed to fully appreciate the joys of life.

Key Words

ANABOLIC STEROIDS: Any synthetic derivative of the hormone testosterone; known to have dangerous side effects.

DISTRESS: A term coined by Selye to identify harmful and unpleasant stress.

DYSMENORRHEA: Painful or difficult menstrual periods.

EUSTRESS: A term coined by Selye to identify stressors that enhance performance and healthy living.

HYPOTHERMIA: Heat loss brought on by rapid cooling, energy loss, and exhaustion; can be life threatening.

MENSTRUATION: The monthly flow of blood from the female genital tract; often called the menstrual period.

NICOTINE: An addictive ingredient found only in tobacco.

PROGRESSIVE MUSCLE RELAXATION: A technique to systematically tighten up and relax selected parts of the body; represents a way to ease tension throughout the body.

SECONDARY AMENORRHEA: Cessation of the menses for a period of at least three to six months.

STRESS: A mental, emotional, and/or physical response to some external demand or event in your life.

WINDCHILL FACTOR: The cooling effect of low temperature and the wind on exposed skin.

A Way of Life Library

Conviser, J., J. Conviser, and H. Harrison. "ACOG's New Exercise Guidelines." *Fitness Management* (April 1994): 38–39.

Hyatt, G. *Exercise and Osteoporosis.* Tucson, AZ: Desert Southwest Fitness, 1995.

Melpomene Institute for Women's Health Research. *The Bodywise Woman.* Champaign, IL: Human Kinetics, 1990.

Williams, M. H. *Beyond Training: How Athletes Enhance Performance Legally and Illegally.* Champaign, IL: Human Kinetics, 1989.

YMCA of the USA with P. Sammann. *YMCA Healthy Back Book.* Champaign, IL: Human Kinetics, 1994.

CHAPTER 13

A *Lifetime of Sports Participation*

It is often assumed that playing sports is a way of improving your level of physical fitness. However, you should play sports for fun, not for fitness. The top athletes are physically fit because they train vigorously. Both amateur and professional athletes commonly devote a significant block of time to training and conditioning. They engage in flexibility, cardiorespiratory, and weight training programs in the off-season (and to a lesser extent during the season) to better prepare themselves for actually playing their sport. The same holds true for the average sports participant: You need to get in shape to play sports, not play sports to get in shape. Good flexibility, cardiorespiratory endurance, and muscular strength and endurance allow a higher level of play and improve your chances of avoiding injury. Although regular sports participation may offer some fitness benefits, do not rely solely on sports to provide you with well-balanced physical fitness.

As you read this chapter, keep these statements in mind:

- The idea that you can play yourself into good physical condition is not supported by research. Most sports need to be supplemented with some basic conditioning.
- The fitness benefits gained from sports participation vary from one person to the next. Factors such as your level of skill, the intensity of the sport, and

the regularity with which you play your chosen sport determine the possible fitness benefits.

- Lifetime sports such as running, swimming, bicycling, and cross-country skiing involve continuous and rhythmical exercise for a sustained period of time and provide a good stimulus to your cardiorespiratory system. Sports such as tennis, racquetball, badminton, gymnastics, and ice skating, although somewhat intermittent activities, can also provide a good total body stimulus if performed vigorously at a high level of skill.

- People often limit themselves in their sports selection. Many physical education programs in schools, colleges, and community fitness centers now offer a wide variety of activities. By sampling new activities, you open up new possibilities for a lifetime of enjoyable sports participation.

Throughout this book, we have described the health benefits of being fit. However, most of us need another reason besides health to motivate us to exercise. Not surprisingly, people who regularly run, cycle, swim, and play sports do so because they enjoy it. Such activities provide the incentive to keep in shape. The more interesting and meaningful a fitness activity or sport is, the greater your chances of involvement and success.

Because we all possess different personalities and interests, we need to select sports and physical activities that meet our own interests and desires. However, this is often easier said than done, simply because many people lack adequate information for making a choice. This chapter provides an overview of a variety of sports activities in which you can get involved for a lifetime of fun and fitness.

A Look at Sports and Physical Fitness

The various sports contribute to physical fitness in different ways. Some sports, such as competitive swimming and cycling, place great stress on the heart and lungs. Weight lifting challenges the muscles and helps to increase muscular strength and endurance. Activities such as karate and gymnastics contribute more to flexibility and strength than do bowling and archery. The physical fitness contributions of different sports are varied and, in some cases, very specific and limited.

For years, many physical education teachers, coaches, and even athletes have operated under the mistaken notion that you can play yourself into good physical condition. This thesis sounds reasonable, but we now know that basic conditioning is needed to supplement most sports programs. You should con-

> **WAY OF LIFE**
> **Considerations When Selecting Lifetime Sports**
>
> - The ability to learn the sport
> - The fitness and skill required to play
> - The potential for injury
> - The initial and recurring costs
> - The time needed to play
>
> - Seasonal limitations
> - The availability of facilities and equipment
> - The fitness and health benefits
> - The sociability and enjoyment potential

dition yourself first to better prepare yourself to play your sport. Possessing adequate levels of flexibility, cardiorespiratory endurance, and muscular strength and endurance will help prevent unnecessary injury and, most important, will increase your enjoyment of your sport.

Getting the Most Out of Sports

Most sports, team or individual, do not provide sufficient continuous rhythmical movement to develop and maintain cardiorespiratory endurance. But regular participation in some sports complements your fitness conditioning program. Sports that require speed and athletic skill provide an important dimension in all-around fitness development. The movements required in the racquet sports, such as badminton, tennis, racquetball, and squash, are excellent for at least maintaining fitness while developing agility, balance, and coordination.

As a general rule, the longer and more continuously a sport is played, the greater the cardiorespiratory benefits. In contrast, sports involving short bursts of movement followed by varying periods of rest do little to develop cardiorespiratory endurance. This point is illustrated by studying the maximal oxygen uptakes (aerobic capacities) of accomplished athletes in different sports. Long-distance runners, cross-country skiers, swimmers, and other endurance athletes have significantly higher average scores (70 to 80 ml/kg/min.) than do football or baseball players, gymnasts, and other top athletes from sports characterized by short bouts of explosive play. In fact, the latter group of athletes have average maximal oxygen uptake values of approximately 50 ml/kg/min.—only slightly above the average for nonathletes. Players of sports that demand a combination of fitness components (short bursts as well as continuous and rhythmical exertions), such as soccer, field hockey, basketball, and tennis, have oxygen uptake values in the high 50s to low 60s.

Rating the Fitness Potential of Lifetime Sports

The benefits of sports participation vary from person to person. Any attempt to rate and compare the sports in terms of their relative contribution to developing physical fitness has limited value. To date, there is only limited research to support such ratings. The intensity of a player's activity and the energy required varies according to age, skill, and fitness level and, in some sports, according to the skill of other players. Therefore the energy cost values for spe-

TABLE 13.1
Fitness Potential of Popular Sports

Sport	Cardiorespiratory Endurance	Muscular Strength and Endurance	
		Upper Body	Lower Body
Backpacking*	Good to fair	Fair	Good
Badminton	Good to fair	Fair	Fair
Baseball/softball	Fair to poor	Fair	Fair
Basketball	Good	Fair	Good
Bowling	Poor	Fair	Poor
Canoeing	Good to fair	Good	Poor
Football (touch)	Fair to poor	Fair	Fair
Golf	Poor	Fair	Good
Handball	Good	Good	Good
Karate	Fair	Good	Good
Racquetball	Good	Good	Good
Scuba diving	Poor	Fair	Fair
Skating (ice)	Good to fair	Poor	Good to fair
Skating (roller)	Good to fair	Poor	Good to fair
Skiing (alpine)	Fair	Good	Good
Skiing (nordic)	Excellent to good	Good	Excellent
Soccer	Good to excellent	Fair	Good to fair
Surfing†	Good†	Good	Good
Tennis	Good to fair	Good to fair	Good
Volleyball	Good to fair	Fair	Good to fair
Waterskiing	Poor	Good	Good

*Benefits depend on the walking terrain and the weight of pack.
†Paddling the board out beyond the breaking waves can be demanding.

cific sports are not as precise as we would like. Still it is valuable to have some basis for comparing the fitness potential of various sports. Table 13.1 lists the fitness potential and energy cost ratings for various sports based on our own as well as others' research. For each sport, a MET range and a range of estimated caloric values is provided. The exact amount of energy (calories) used depends on how much you weigh (heavier individuals expend more calories) and on how vigorously you play. Terms that qualify the overall potential of each sport to develop fitness (excellent, good, fair, poor) are also provided to help you to make comparisons. What is most important is how demanding these sports are

TABLE 13.1				
Fitness Potential of Popular Sports (continued)				
Sport	**Flexibility**	**MET Range**	**Calories per Minute**	**Caloric Range (Cal hr.)**
Backpacking*	Fair	4–8	5–10	300–600
Badminton	Fair	4–8	5–10	300–600
Baseball/softball	Fair	3–6	4–7.5	240–450
Basketball	Fair	8–10	10–12.5	600–750
Bowling	Poor	2–3	2.5–4	150–240
Canoeing	Poor	3–8	4–10	240–600
Football (touch)	Fair	4–8	5–10	300–600
Golf	Fair	3–4	4–5	240–300
Handball	Fair	6–12	10–12.5	600–750
Karate	Excellent	6–8	7.5–10	450–600
Racquetball	Fair	6–10	7.5–12.5	450–750
Scuba diving	Fair	4–6	5–7.5	300–450
Skating (ice)	Fair	4–8	5–10	300–600
Skating (roller)	Fair	4–8	5–10	300–600
Skiing (alpine)	Good	5–9	6–10	360–600
Skiing (nordic)	Good	6–12	7.5–15	450–900
Soccer	Good	6–12	7.5–15	450–900
Surfing[†]	Good	4–10	5–12.5	300–750
Tennis	Fair	4–8	5–10	300–600
Volleyball	Fair	4–8	5–10	300–600
Waterskiing	Fair	4–6	5–7.5	300–450

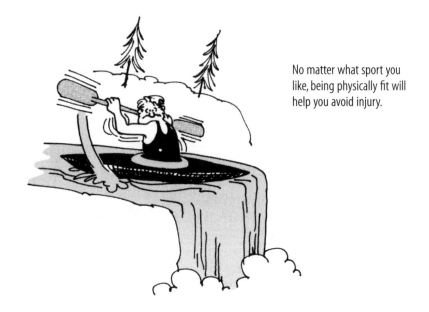

No matter what sport you like, being physically fit will help you avoid injury.

on the body. In other words, what are the specific physiological requirements of each?

For example, let's look at racquetball. It is a sport that most people can play with reasonable success after brief instruction and practice. How does it rate as a fitness activity? Racquetball is vigorous, it uses large muscle groups, it requires high levels of energy, and it is generally played for at least an hour. It is played not continuously but intermittently, with brief stops between serves. Successful play is highly dependent on the functional ability of your circulatory and aerobic systems. Racquetball requires strength and particularly muscular endurance. The flexibility required is limited to a few muscles and joints. Therefore, as Table 13.1 shows, racquetball rates "good" on cardiorespiratory endurance and on muscular strength and endurance (upper and lower body), and "fair" on flexibility.

Keep in mind that these ratings are based on the average participant, not the expert player. Generally the energy required to play racquetball properly can range from as low as 8 METs to as high as 12 METs. The reason for this wide range is the variance in both the skill and fitness capabilities of the participant. To put it another way, 8 METs, when it represents maximal cardiorespiratory endurance, is considered low. One needs a 10- or 11-MET maximum to be able to perform an activity at an 8-MET level. On the other end of the scale, if you are capable of playing racquetball at a 12-MET level, you would need a 15- to 16-MET maximum. This example further underscores the point that you need to get in shape if you want to play your favorite sport to your fullest capability. The better your physical condition, the better your chance of getting a good workout when playing sports. If you presently possess a low level of fitness, investing significant amounts of time playing racquetball or any other sport to develop fitness is probably not worthwhile. First, involve your total body in a well-rounded program to develop your heart, lungs, and muscles; then you can fully enjoy the maximal benefits of sports participation.

Now let's look at golf. After spending over two years studying the fitness and energy responses of people who play golf, researchers at the University of Illinois concluded that golf is not a suitable activity for developing fitness. They compared 20 middle-aged male golfers and similar control groups of nongolfers and runners (running 8 to 12 miles per week) on over 30 fitness measures. The control group and the golfers were very inactive prior to the golf season, when they were first tested. When retested in early September, each golfer felt he was in better shape, but when compared to the control group, the golfers showed improvement in only one meaure—leg strength. Cardiorespiratory measures did not improve; those in the running group were still far superior to the golfers. Extensive energy-cost studies were also done on four of the golfers. The results showed the average energy requirement for golf to be about three times that of sitting in a chair (3 METs). As this study indicated, the exercise

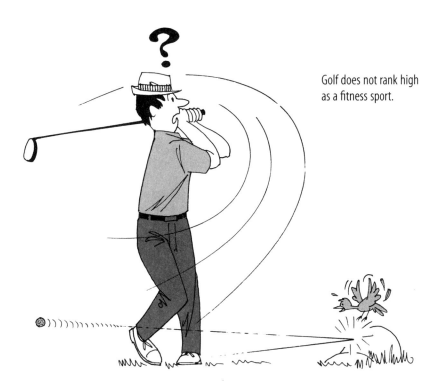

Golf does not rank high as a fitness sport.

WAY OF LIFE
What Lifetime Sports Can Offer

- A reason to stay in shape
- Excitement and challenge
- A sense of accomplishment
- Friendships and social opportunities
- Fun!

requirements of golf, in terms of both energy cost and heart-rate stimulation, are not adequate for fitness gains. Since this study was conducted, other researchers have come up with similar findings.

Summary

Throughout this book, we have emphasized the importance of following a regular schedule (three times a week at least) of vigorous health-promoting exercise. The availability of facilities is just one of the problems involved in establishing a regular routine for playing sports for fitness. A simple handball match can be complicated by details such as reserving a court, finding an opponent, and setting a time that fits your schedule. If you choose a seasonal outdoor sport, bad weather can spoil the best-made plans. Most sports are not suitable for daily or three-times-a-week programs. Still, they can provide a welcome break from your regular workouts.

Now is the time to begin developing skills and interests in sports that you can play in the years to come. University and college physical education programs around the country now provide instruction in many lifetime sports. Take advantage of the opportunity to enroll in these classes. Don't shy away from unfamiliar sports. All sports have exciting and challenging qualities that make them fun and popular. Activities such as skiing, karate, ice-skating, sailing, and orienteering reflect the variety of offerings now found in college curriculums. And don't forget that running, cycling, and swimming (the cardiorespiratory developers) are also lifetime sports. Fun runs, road races, triathlons, and cycling tours are enjoyed by people of all ages.

Finally, participating in sports is another way to enjoy the pleasures of being physically fit. Physical fitness is a way of life. Good luck!

GLOSSARY

AEROBIC CAPACITY / VO$_2$MAX: The greatest amount of oxygen that you can consume per minute; a functional measure of your physical fitness.

AEROBICS: A variety of vigorous exercise routines and activities performed to music.

AMINO ACIDS: The end product of the breakdown of protein.

ANABOLIC STEROIDS: Any synthetic derivative of the hormone testosterone; known to have dangerous side effects.

ARTERIOSCLEROSIS: The advanced stage of atherosclerosis when the arteries become hardened.

ATHEROSCLEROSIS: A condition in which the deposits of fatty substances on the inner walls of the arteries build up, narrowing the blood vessels.

ATHLETIC SKILL/MOTOR ABILITY: The ability of muscles to function harmoniously and efficiently, resulting in smooth, coordinated muscular movement; a reflection of general athletic skill.

BALLISTIC STRETCHING: A technique for increasing flexibility that involves bouncing and momentum; generally not recommended for the average fitness participant.

BASAL METABOLIC RATE (BMR): The minimal level of energy required to sustain life at complete rest.

BLOOD SUGAR: The glucose found in the blood which is used for energy or stored as glycogen in cells.

BODYBUILDING: A type of exercise program designed specifically to cause as much muscle enlargement as possible. Bodybuilding is also a sport in which the competitors are judged on muscle development and symmetry.

BODY COMPOSITION: The relative amounts of fat and lean body tissue (such as muscle and bone) that make up one's body.

CALORIE: A unit of measure for the rate of heat or energy production in the body from food; often called a kilocalorie.

CARBOHYDRATES: A food substance that is the primary energy food for vigorous muscular activity; includes various sugars and starches and is found in the body in the form of glucose and glycogen.

CARDIAC OUTPUT: The amount of blood pumped in 1 minute by the heart.

CARDIAC REHABILITATION: The management of patients after open-heart surgery or heart attack through a program of exercise and other related interventions to restore their capacity to live meaningful and healthy lives.

CARDIORESPIRATORY ENDURANCE: The capacity of the heart, blood vessels, and lungs to function efficiently during vigorous, sustained activity such as running, swimming, or cycling.

CHOLESTEROL: The waxy, fattylike substance that functions as a building block in forming compounds that are vital to body functions. It is produced in the body and is also obtained by eating foods of animal origin. Elevated levels of cholesterol in the blood have been associated with an increased risk of heart and blood vessel disease.

CONCENTRIC ACTION: A type of muscle action in which force is generated while the muscle shortens. Concentric muscle actions are performed during the up-phase of a lift.

CONDITIONING PERIOD: The portion of a workout in which the body is vigorously exercised. The conditioning period can consist of any physically challenging activity as long as the frequency, intensity, and duration are sufficient to cause a training response.

COOL-DOWN: The last element of a workout consisting of a tapering-off in exercise intensity. The cool-down should include light general-type activity along with stretching exercises.

CORONARY HEART DISEASE: The impairment of the coronary arteries to deliver blood due to a buildup of cholesterol and associated fatty substances on the inner portion of the artery walls.

CROSS-TRAINING: A training practice in which a variety of different exercise activities are used to accomplish fitness goals.

DIABETES: A chronic disorder of glucose (sugar) metabolism due to a disturbance in the normal insulin mechanism.

DIASTOLIC BLOOD PRESSURE: The lowest force exerted by the arterial blood flow against the walls of the vessels.

DISTRESS: A term coined by Selye to identify harmful and unpleasant stress.

DURATION: A training variable associated with the overload principle that denotes the length of the workout session. The duration of a workout varies depending on the type of training being performed.

DYNAMIC EXERCISES: Exercises that involve joint movement.

DYSMENORRHEA: Painful or difficult menstrual periods.

ECCENTRIC ACTION: A type of muscle action in which force is generated while the muscle lengthens. Eccentric muscle actions are performed during the lowering phase of a lift.

ENERGY EXPENDITURE: The energy released during exercise; often referred to as caloric cost.

EUSTRESS: A term coined by Selye to identify stressors that enhance performance and healthy living.

EXERCISE ADHERENCE: The practice of closely following a regular exercise program.

EXERCISE HEART RATE: A heart-beat rate (or pulse rate) per minute during exercise that produces significant cardiorespiratory benefits.

EXPLOSIVENESS: A muscle's ability to generate force as quickly as possible.

FAT: A food substance that is a source of energy in the body; an insulator and protector of vital organs.

FAT WEIGHT: The absolute amount of body fat, usually expressed in pounds.

FATTY ACID: The end product of the breakdown of fats in the body.

FIELD TESTS: Tests that take place outside the laboratory.

FLEXIBILITY: The range of movement of a specific joint and its corresponding muscle groups.

FREE WEIGHTS: Equipment such as bars, plate weights, dumbbells, and barbells used in resistance training.

FREQUENCY: A training variable associated with the overload principle that refers to the number of times (usually on a per week basis) training is performed.

GLUCOSE: A type of carbohydrate that is transported in the blood and metabolized in the cell; also called blood sugar.

GLYCOGEN: The storage form of carbohydrates found in the liver and muscles.

HALF-MARATHON: A footrace of 13.1 miles, half the distance of a marathon.

HEALTH: The general condition of one's physical, intellectual, social, emotional, and spiritual being. Health is best depicted as a continuum with death and wellness at its extremes.

HIGH-DENSITY LIPOPROTEIN (HDL) CHOLESTEROL: One of the major classes of lipoprotein, often referred to as HDL cholesterol. High levels of HDL cholesterol are associated with increased protection against heart disease.

HIGH-IMPACT AEROBICS: Aerobics routines involving movements in which both feet may be off the floor at the same time.

HIGH-IMPACT EXERCISE: Endurance activities in which both feet are off the exercise surface at one point or another.

HYPERTENSION: A higher-than-normal blood pressure, usually defined as any systolic pressure at or above 140 mmHg and/or a diastolic pressure at or above 90 mmHg.

HYPOTHERMIA: Heat loss brought on by rapid cooling, energy loss, and exhaustion; can be life threatening.

INDIRECT CALORIMETRY: A method for measuring energy expenditure by relating the heat loss from energy expenditure to the amount of oxygen consumed by the body; it can be used to calculate the number of calories expended during a given activity by determining the amount of oxygen utilized.

INSULIN: A hormone that controls the rate of glucose entry into cells.

INTENSITY: A training variable associated with the overload principle that refers to how difficult the training is. The intensity of a training program is gauged differently depending on the nature of the exercise. For example, cardiorespiratory exercise intensity is determined based on heart rate.

INTERVAL TRAINING: Training made up of successive bouts of exercise at near maximal intensity alternated with periods of rest or lighter exercise such as brisk walking or slow jogging.

ISOMETRIC TRAINING: A mode of resistance training in which the muscles generate force, but with no resulting joint movement.

ISOTONIC TRAINING: A dynamic mode of resistance training in which the muscles generate force against a constant resistance, such as when performing a bench press with an 80-pound barbell.

LEAN BODY WEIGHT: The absolute amount of lean body tissue, usually expressed in pounds. Muscle, bone, and organ tissue make up the majority of lean body tissue.

LIPIDS: Fats, or fatlike substances, such as fatty acids, triglycerides, and cholesterol.

LIPOPROTEIN: A type of protein that carries cholesterol and triglycerides in the bloodstream.

LOW-DENSITY LIPOPROTEIN (LDL) CHOLESTEROL: A carrier of large amounts of fat and cholesterol from the liver, where they are made, to the tissues of the body. This is the cholesterol that accumulates in the arteries and leads to clogged arteries.

LOW-IMPACT AEROBICS: Aerobics routines in which one foot is always in contact with the floor.

LOW-IMPACT EXERCISE: Endurance activities in which one foot always maintains contact with the exercise surface.

MARATHON: A footrace covering 26.2 miles.

MENSTRUATION: The monthly flow of blood from the female genital tract; often called the menstrual period.

MET: The rate of energy expended at rest in 1 minute; used to rate activities in multiples above the resting rate; 3.5 milliliters of oxygen per kilogram body weight per minute.

MINERALS: A group of 22 metallic elements vital to proper cell functioning.

MINI WARM-UP: The additional period of light exercise needed to gradually increase heart and breathing rates and muscle temperature if an exerciser has stopped to stretch after an initial cardiorespiratory endurance exercise warm-up.

MUSCLE FIBER HYPERPLASIA: An increase in the number of cells found within a muscle.

MUSCLE HYPERTROPHY: The enlargement of muscle, usually resulting from resistance training.

MUSCULAR ENDURANCE: The capacity of a muscle to contract repeatedly or to hold a fixed or static contraction over a period of time.

MUSCULAR STRENGTH: The maximal amount of force generated by a muscle or group of muscles.

MYOCARDIAL INFARCTION: Death of part of the heart muscle (myocardium) caused by an interruption of the blood supply to the area; also called a heart attack.

NICOTINE: An addictive ingredient found only in tobacco.

NONIMPACT EXERCISE: Endurance activities without an air-borne phase, in which the exerciser is seated or buoyed by water.

NUTRIENTS: The basic substances needed by the body that are provided by eating food.

NUTRITION: The foods we eat and how our bodies process them.

NUTRITIONAL ERGOGENIC AIDS: Special foods or supplements that are touted to improve physical fitness levels or athletic performance.

OBESITY: The state of being too fat.

OLESTRA: A fat substitute; "fake fat."

OXYGEN UPTAKE: The consumption of oxygen, indicating the amount of energy the body uses; 1 liter of oxygen = 4.8 calories.

PHYSICAL FITNESS: A physiological state blending health-related and skill-related components that reflects the body's ability to meet physical challenges and resist diseases associated with sedentary living.

PLYOMETRICS: Exercises designed to improve one's muscle power or explosiveness.

PROGRESSIVE MUSCLE RELAXATION: A technique to systematically tighten up and relax selected parts of the body; represents a way to ease tension throughout the body.

PROTEIN: A food substance that provides the basic structural components of cells and is also the source for enzymes and hormones in the body.

REPETITION: A single muscle contraction or lift.

REPETITIONS MAXIMUM (RM): The maximum load that can be lifted a given number of times. For example, 6RM refers to the maximum weight that can be lifted six but not seven times.

RISK: The possibility or chance that something will happen. In health, it is often expressed in degrees of danger.

SATURATED FATS: A food source found in meat, whole milk, cheese, and butter; are solid at room temperature.

SECONDARY AMENORRHEA: Cessation of the menses for a period of at least three to six months.

SET: A group of repetitions or lifts performed in succession without rest.

SKINFOLD CALIPERS: An instrument used in body composition assessment to measure the thickness of a fold of skin and its underlying, or subcutaneous, fat.

SPOTTER: A person who assists with safety, checks form, and encourages the lifter performing a resistance exercise.

STATIC STRETCHING: A technique for increasing flexibility that involves holding a position at the point of slight discomfort without using bouncing or jerking motions.

STEP AEROBICS: A low-impact, high-intensity form of aerobics that involves stepping on and off a bench ranging in height from 4 to 12 inches using a variety of step and arm combinations.

STRENGTH TRAINING: An exercise program that is designed specifically to increase muscular strength.

STRESS: A mental, emotional, and/or physical response to some external demand or event in your life.

SUGAR: A term often misused; in this book it refers to refined sugar or table sugar. The scientific name for sugar is sucrose.

SYSTOLIC BLOOD PRESSURE: The greatest force exerted by the arterial blood flow against the walls of the vessels.

TARGET HEART-RATE RANGE: The range in heart rate necessary to achieve cardiorespiratory overload and subsequent improvement in cardiorespiratory endurance; 50 to 85 percent of heart-rate reserve, according to the American College of Sports Medicine.

10-PERCENT PROGRAM: An easy and safe rule of thumb to follow concerning weekly increases in duration in cardiorespiratory endurance training.

TEST BATTERY: A series of tests used to measure the various components of physical fitness.

TRAINING EFFECT: Gradual improvements to the exercised heart, lungs, and muscles that allow them to function at a higher level both during physical exertion and at rest.

TRAINING HEART RATE: A heart-beat rate (or pulse rate) per minute during exercise that produces significant cardiorespiratory benefits.

TRIATHLON: A competitive event involving three endurance-type activities such as swimming, cycling, and running.

TRIGLYCERIDES: The most common form of fat found in the body; composed of three fatty acids.

TYPE A BEHAVIOR: Behaviors such as an excessive competitive drive and a sense of urgency about time that tend to predispose one to heart disease.

UNSATURATED FATS: A liquid type of fat found in peanut oil and olive oil.

VALSALVA MANEUVER: The act of holding one's breath, often when lifting weights. The Valsalva maneuver causes dangerous fluctuations in blood pressure and should be avoided.

VITAMINS: Organic substances that perform vital functions within the cells.

WARM-UP: The beginning element of a workout that prepares your body for more vigorous exercise. Generally walking and stretching of the major muscle groups are done during the warm-up period.

WATER AEROBICS: An offshoot of land-based aerobics; performed in a swimming pool.

WEIGHT-BEARING EXERCISE: Endurance activities in which one or both feet maintain contact with the ground and support the body.

WEIGHT LIFTER'S BLACKOUT: Passing out during weight lifting due to performing the Valsalva maneuver (breath holding).

WELLNESS: The state of health that results when physical, intellectual, spiritual, social, and emotional components are all at optimal levels.

WINDCHILL FACTOR: The cooling effect of low temperature and the wind on exposed skin.

INDEX